SPORTS
PHYSICAL
THERAPY

CLINICS IN PHYSICAL THERAPY VOLUME 10

EDITORIAL BOARD

Otto D. Payton, Ph.D., **Chairman**

Louis R. Amundsen, Ph.D.

Suzann K. Campbell, Ph.D.

Jules M. Rothstein, Ph.D.

Already Published

SPORTS PHYSICAL THERAPY

Edited by

Donna B. Bernhardt
M.S., R.P.T., A.T.C.

Assistant Professor
Department of Physical Therapy
Boston University–Sargent College of Allied
  Health Professions
Boston, Massachusetts

CHURCHILL LIVINGSTONE
NEW YORK, EDINBURGH, LONDON, MELBOURNE
1986

Library of Congress Cataloging-in-Publication Data
Main entry under title:

Sports physical therapy.

  (Clinics in physical therapy ; v. 10)
  Includes bibliographies and index.
  1. Sports—Physiological aspects. 2. Sports—
Accidents and injuries. I. Bernhardt, Donna B.
II. Title. [DNLM; 1. Physical Therapy. 2. Sports
Medicine. W1 CL831CN v.10 / QT 260 S78565]
RC1235.S664 1986   617'.1027   85-31335
ISBN 0-443-08444-0

Distributed in the United Kingdom by Churchill Livingstone, Robert
Stevenson House, 1–3 Baxter's Place, Leith Walk, Edinburgh EH1
3AF, and by associated companies, branches, and representatives
throughout the world.

Accurate indications, adverse reactions, and dosage schedules for
drugs are provided in this book, but it is possible that they may
change. The reader is urged to review the package information data of
the manufacturers of the medications mentioned.

Acquisitions Editor: *Kim Loretucci*
Copy Editor: *Anne L. Kellogg*
Production Designer: *Charlie Lebeda*
Production Supervisor: *Jane Grochowski*

Printed in the United States of America

First published in 1986

Contributors

Lawrence E. Armstrong, Ph.D.
Research Physiologist, Heat Research, U.S. Army Research Institute of Environmental Medicine, Natick, Massachusetts

Mary Bauman, R.D.
Department of Health Sciences—Nutrition, Boston University–Sargent College of Allied Health Professions, Boston, Massachusetts

Donna B. Bernhardt, M.S., R.P.T., A.T.C.
Assistant Professor, Department of Physical Therapy, Boston University–Sargent College of Allied Health Professions, Boston, Massachusetts

William L. Daniels, Ph.D.
Exercise Physiology Division, U.S. Army Research Institute of Environmental Medicine, Natick, Massachusetts

John M. Davis, B.S., L.P.T., A.T.C.
Physical Therapist, Division of Sports Medicine, University of North Carolina; Head Trainer, Basketball Team, University of North Carolina, Chapel Hill, North Carolina

Joseph E. Dziados, M.D.
Research Medical Officer, Exercise Physiology Division, U.S. Army Research Institute of Environmental Medicine, Natick, Massachusetts

Jeffrey E. Falkel, Ph.D., L.P.T.
Assistant Professor of Physical Therapy and Physiology, Department of Physical Therapy, Ohio University, Athens, Ohio

Janet E. Guilfoyle, M.S., A.T.C.
Instructor, Department of Health, Sport, and Leisure Studies, Northeastern University, Boston Bouvé College, Boston, Massachusetts

William J. Kraemer, Ph.D.
Exercise Physiology Division, U.S. Army Research Institute of Environmental Medicine, Natick, Massachusetts

John S. Leard, M.Ed., P.P.T., A.T.C.
Athletic Trainer/Physical Therapist, Lane Health Center, Northeastern University; Lecturer, Department of Health, Sport, and Leisure Studies, Northeastern University, Boston Bouvé College, Boston, Massachusetts

Barney F. LeVeau, Ph.D.
Professor and Chairman, Department of Physical Therapy, University of Texas Health Science Center at Dallas, School of Allied Health Sciences, Dallas, Texas

Robert G. McMurray, Ph.D.
Associate Professor of Physical Education and Director, Human Performance Laboratory, Physical Education Department, University of North Carolina; Associate Professor of Physical Therapy, Division of Allied Health Sciences, University of North Carolina, Chapel Hill, North Carolina

David Yukelson, Ph.D.
Sports Psychologist and Administrative Manager, Hermann Hospital Center for Sports Medicine, Houston; Adjunct Professor, Department of HPER, University of Houston; Clinical Instructor, Department of Pediatrics, University of Texas Medical School at Houston, Houston, Texas

Preface

The specialty area of sports medicine is relatively new and nebulously defined. Yet, if one considers this medical specialty as the total care of the athlete, it becomes an extremely broad field that demands a tremendous breadth as well as depth of knowledge.

Each athlete should be treated as a whole person. All aspects of the athlete's physiology and function must be addressed. Care encompasses prevention, conditioning, training, and rehabilitation.

The intent of this volume is to provide a general, but clinically applicable overview of the care of the athlete for the health care professional or student who intervenes with an occasional athlete. Clear awareness and understanding of all aspects of care are vital for effective intervention. Additionally, knowledge is the keystone of trust for the athlete in any health care provider; thus, a firm knowledge base assumes great importance.

Each chapter addresses the effects of exercise and sport on the various systems of the organism. The physiological responses to exercise in both the untrained and trained individual are outlined. The effects of warm up–cool down, nutrition, training protocols, and the environment are discussed. Injury—the biomechanics and immediate and long-term care—are presented theoretically as an intervention model. Finally, the psychology of sport and athletic participation are discussed.

The authors hope to impart an interesting and informative basis for care of the sportsperson. The volume brought together some of the best minds in the field of sports medicine to produce very meaningful and enjoyable results.

Donna B. Bernhardt, M.S., R.P.T., A.T.C.

Contents

SPORTS
PHYSICAL
THERAPY

1 | Examination of the Integrated Physiological Responses and Mechanisms During Exercise

Robert G. McMurray

The study of exercise physiology centers on the events involved with skeletal muscle contraction. All other physiological systems (cardiovascular, respiratory, endocrine, renal, and thermoregulatory) operate to support the muscle's function and the individual's integrity. The link between the physiological systems is most evident between the respiratory, cardiovascular, and muscular systems. Oxygen, absorbed in the lungs, is transported to the working muscle via the cardiovascular system. Any compromise in either the cardiovascular or respiratory systems will reduce the capacity of the muscle to contract, ultimately limiting exercise. Such a response is most noticeable in patients with cardiovascular disease or obstructive lung disease. Because the physiological responses to exercise are so closely interrelated, I first discuss the basic systemic responses to exercise, then relate the systems as their responses would occur from the onset of exercise, through a steady state, and into exhaustion.

ENERGY FOR MUSCLE CONTRACTION

Energy for muscle contraction is obtained from two major pathways: anaerobic (without oxygen) and aerobic (with oxygen). During exercise the choice of the dominant pathway is dependent on the intensity and duration of exercise. Adenosine triphosphate (ATP) is the only high-energy compound that is the source of energy for all muscle contractions. ATP is broken down into adenosine diphosphate (ADP) and an inorganic phosphate; in the process, energy for muscle contraction is produced. The resting skeletal muscle contains enough ATP for only a few twitches. Small amounts of cellular ATP may be an advantage as energy production is controlled by the cellular ATP:ADP ratio.[1] Therefore, any small reduction in ATP would initiate energy production. The muscle cell also has a secondary source of energy: creatine phosphate (CP). CP stores high-energy phosphate and can give up this energy to ADP to form more ATP via the following reaction[2]:

$$CP \rightarrow C + P + energy$$

$$ADP + Pi + energy \rightarrow ATP$$

This reaction takes place in the sarcoplasm of the muscle cell without the presence of oxygen and provides enough energy for a 100-m sprint (10 to 15 seconds). Since few chemical reactions are involved, the energy can be provided very quickly. Fox[3] suggested that the ATP–CP stores provide only 0.7 mol of ATP but can provide it at a rate of 3.6 mol/minute. CP has also been associated with the aerobic pathways as a shuttle for transporting the energy formed in the mitochondria to the ADP in the sarcomeres (contractile units).[4]

Anaerobic Energy Pathway: Glycolysis

Although the ATP–CP energy pathway is considered anaerobic, the main anaerobic pathway involves the breakdown of glycogen or glucose to pyruvic acid[2]: "glycolysis" (Fig. 1-1). Pyruvic acid is then converted to lactic acid with the assistance of an enzyme M-lactate dehydrogenase (M-LDH). In this 11-step process, glucose or glycogen is phosphatized, converted to a phosphatized fructose, then converted to two phosphatized three-carbon carboxylic acids (pyruvic acid). ATP is used to phosphatize the sugars, but it is produced in larger quantities than used, for a net gain of two ATP per single glucose or three ATP per single glycogen used. Glycolysis also produces a reduced nucleotide (NADH2), which during anaerobiosis donates the hydrogens to pyruvic acid for the formation of lactic acid. NADH2 can be used as energy for the aerobic pathway when sufficient oxygen is present. Glycolysis has been considered an "inefficient" energy system because the net energy gain is small and it also produces lactic acid, which, when accumulated, slows and ultimately stops energy metabolism. The benefit of the system is that it provides energy at a fairly high rate, higher than the aerobic pathways. Fox[3] suggested that

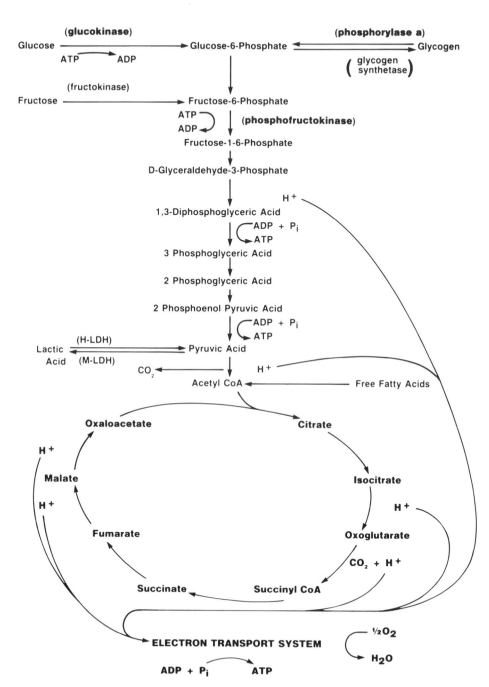

Fig. 1-1. Schematic representation of the anaerobic and aerobic energy production pathways.

Table 1-1. Aerobic Energy Production

Process	Energy Produced (ATP)
Glycolysis (-2 ATP $+$ 4 ATP)	2
Krebs' cycle (1 ATP $\times$ 2 acetyl-CoA)	2
Electron transport system	
Oxidation of FADH2 (2 ATP/FADH $\times$ 2)	4
Oxidation of NADH2 (3 ATP/NADH $\times$ 10)	30
Total	38

From data in references 1, 6–8, and 9.

glycolysis produces about 1.2 mol of energy at a production rate of 1.6 mol/minute, but more recent evidence[1] suggests that the total capacity is greater.

The largest portion of lactic acid produced during anaerobic glycolysis is used directly as a source of energy, if sufficient oxygen is present.[1] In the skeletal and heart muscles an enzyme, H-lactate dehydrogenase (H-LDH), converts lactic acid to pyruvic acid (Fig. 1-1), which is then broken down to CO_2 and water via the aerobic energy pathway. Thus energy is directly formed. Lactate also can be transported back to the liver, where it enters the Cori cycle: it is converted to glycogen and then to glucose to replenish blood glucose stores (essentially the reverse of glycolysis). The metabolism of lactate was believed to be responsible for the elevation of the metabolic rate after the cessation of exercise (oxygen debt). Recent evidence[5] suggests that the lactate actually plays only a minor role and that other factors, such as temperature, hormones, energy for respiration and heart, myoglobin, and replenishing ATP–CP stores, are more important.

Aerobic Pathway: Oxidative Phosphorylation

Pyruvic acid and lactic acid have considerable amounts of energy stored within their chemical bonds, but oxygen must be present to release this energy for the production of ATP. This process takes place in the aerobic pathway (Fig. 1-1). In the presence of oxygen, the pyruvic acid formed in the sarcoplasm during glycolysis enters the mitochondria and is broken down to acetyl-CoA and CO_2. The acetyl-CoA enters the Krebs' cycle (citric acid cycle), in which it is dismantled to supply hydrogen ions and electrons to the cytochrome chain (electron transport system) for energy production. The nucleotides NAD and FAD are used to transport the energy to the electron transport system. In the electron transport system, the electrons and hydrogen ions from glycolysis and the Krebs' cycle are transported through six carrier compounds and ultimately combine with oxygen to form water. During the transportation process, chemical energy is released. This energy is used to combine ADP and Pi to form ATP. One molecule of acetyl-CoA entering the Krebs' cycle will produce one ATP in the Krebs' cycle and 17 ATPs in the electron transport system. Therefore, the total energy production from one molecule of glucose is 38 ATPs (Table 1-1).[1,2,4] When one molecule of glycogen is used as the source of energy, the total energy production is 39 ATPs.[4] The process of converting glucose to glycogen involves the phosphorylation of the glucose molecule, which uses one ATP. Since this step has been already completed, glycogen entering the glycolytic pathway uses only one ATP during the catabolism, yet four ATPs are produced. This increase in efficiency and the ease of accessibility are two reasons why glycogen is preferred to glucose during strenuous exertion.

Fats are also used as a source of energy. Fats are stored in the adipose tissue and skeletal muscles in the form of triglycerides. Triglycerides are broken down to free fatty acids (FFA) and glycerol by the enzyme lipase. FFA enters beta oxidation, a five-step reaction in which two carbon chains are cleaved, or lysed,[2] and changed to acetyl-CoA, which enters the Krebs' cycle following the aerobic pathway as glucose or glycogen (Fig. 1-1). Because one molecule of FFA is larger than one molecule of glucose, more energy, per molecule of FFA is formed, but the process is slower. The glycerol formed in the breakdown of triglycerides goes through a three-step process, entering glycolysis at an intermediate step, and therefore also can be used as energy.

Proteins also can be a source of energy, but they are utilized only to a minor degree in nonfasting persons. Evans and associates[10] estimated that protein accounts for only 5.5 percent of the energy used during exercise. Proteins are first broken down into amino acids, then enter into glycolysis or the Krebs' cycle at the appropriate site. For example, alanine is converted to pyruvic acid and isolucine is transformed to succinate, an intermediate in the Krebs' cycle. Amino acids also can enter the liver and undergo the process of gluconeogenesis to increase blood glucose levels.[2] This process usually occurs during exercise under the control of the hormone glucagon.[11,12]

Regardless of the choice of substrate for the production of ATP, the aerobic energy pathway has the capacity to sustain exercise for prolonged periods of time. In a normal human, the aerobic systems can produce more than 150 mol of ATP, but they produce it at a maximal rate of only 1 mol/minute. Since respiration and cardiac output must increase to provide the oxygen for the aerobic pathway, this pathway takes a few minutes to reach peak efficiency.

Control of Energy Metabolism

There are several controls that determine the choice of metabolic pathway and fuel.[2,13] The ATP:ADP ratio affects both the anaerobic and aerobic pathways. When ATP stores are reduced (ATP < ADP), creatine phosphate breakdown is activated and the activity of the key enzymes of glycogen utilization (phosphorylase) and glycolysis (phosphofructokinase) is enhanced. As the mitochondrial ADP increases, the aerobic pathway is activated. Oxygen availability is another controlling factor in energy metabolism. When sufficient oxygen is present to convert pyruvic acid to acetyl-CoA, the aerobic pathway dominates. Fat requires more oxygen to catabolize than sugars; therefore abundant oxygen must be available to utilize fats. When oxygen is at a premium or inadequate to convert substantial amounts of pyruvic acid to acetyl-CoA, pyruvic acid forms lactic acid, which, in turn, blocks beta oxidation and enhances glycolysis[13-15] (unless the acid buildup is too great, diminishing all metabolism).

Citrate, an intermediate compound in the Krebs' cycle, affects glycolysis: an increase in citrate causes a deactivation of glucokinase, phosphorylase, and phosphofructokinase, reducing glucose and glycogen utilization as well as glycolysis. An increase in calcium activates glycolysis, and a decrease in calcium has the reverse effect.[1] Elevated catecholamines, particularly epinephrine, enhance energy metabolism.[1,2] Epinephrine activates glucokinse, phosphorylase, and phosphofructokinase, thus increasing glycolysis. It also activates lipase, which increases FFA in the blood. Of course, the source of fuel substrate is ultimately related to availability. If only fats and protein are available, then FFA catabolism is enhanced. If glucose, fats, and proteins are available, the dominant source of energy depends on oxygen availability. Generally, the body attempts to supply all the energy via the aerobic pathway. When the aerobic system is incapable of meeting the energy demands, the anaerobic system is used.

The level of activity of the aerobic pathway can be determined by measuring the oxygen uptake. In the production of energy, the aerobic pathway utilizes oxygen to form carbon dioxide and water. Therefore, the more oxygen used, the greater the use of the aerobic pathway. The measurement of maximal oxygen uptake is at present the best available indicator of cardiovascular fitness. (Tables of norms are available in most exercise, physiology, and fitness textbooks).[4,6] If the person is not in a starvation state, CO_2 production can be measured to find an indication of substrate utilization. Close examination of glucose metabolism indicates that for each molecule completely catabolized, six oxygen molecules are used and six carbon dioxides are produced: a $CO_2:O_2$ ratio of 1.0. In contrast, if 13 carbon FFA is catabolized, 23 molecules of oxygen are used but only 16 carbon dioxides are produced: a $CO_2:O_2$ ratio of about 0.7. This ratio is called the R value.[1,2,4,6] The R value for protein is approximately 0.85. Since protein plays such a minor role in exercise metabolism it is at present discounted and the R value used as an indicator of either fat or carbohydrate metabolism. Given the R value, the number of calories used for the activity can be determined. If the R value is 1.0, indicating glucose utilization, then for every liter of oxygen consumed, 5.047 kcals of energy is produced. When FFAs are the primary source of energy, with an R value of 0.70, the energy equivalent is only 4.686 kcals. Tables for the caloric equivalent per liter of oxygen at any nonprotein R value are available in most standard exercise physiology texts.[4,6] The caloric energy expenditure of the activity is determined by multiplying the oxygen uptake (in L/minute) by the amount of energy produced (kcals/L of O_2).

MUSCLE

Three types of skeletal muscle fibers exist[7]: slow-twitch (type 1), fast-twitch oxidative (type 2a), and fast-twitch glycolytic (type 2b). The slow twitch type 1 fibers have a contraction time of approximately 110 ms, and type 2b

Table 1-2. Characteristics of Human Skeletal Muscle Fiber Types

Characteristic	Slow-twitch (Type 1)	Fast-twitch Type 2a	Fast-twitch Type 2b
Size	Small	Intermediate	Large
Myosin ATPase activity	Low	Moderate	High
Sarcoplasmic reticulum	Poor	Great	Great
Force produced	Small	Intermediate	Large
Fatigability	Slight	Moderate	Extremely
Mitochondria	Many	Moderate	Few
Aerobic enzymes	Many	Moderate[a]	Few
Triglyceride stores	Large	Moderate	Low
Capillaries	Many	Moderate	Few
Myoglobin content	High	High	Low
Glycolytic capacity	Poor	Moderate[a]	Great
Glycogen stores	Low	Moderate[a]	High
ATP–CP stores	Low	Moderate[a]	High

[a] The quantity is dependent on physical training.

fibers take about 50 ms to contract.[16] Type 2a fibers contract not quite as fast as type 2b fibers. Type 1 slow twitch fibers are smaller than fast-twitch fibers and produce less force, but they are more energy-efficient and quite fatigue-resistant. Vrbova[17] noted that fast-twitch fibers (type 2) contain much more myosin ATPase, an enzyme necessary for energy liberation for muscle contraction. Differences in the molecular structure of the myosin and myosin ATPase of the slow- and fast-twitch fibers affect the speed of contraction.[1] Also, slow-twitch fibers (type 1) have a more poorly developed sarcoplasmic reticulum, resulting in a reduced rate of calcium release. Calcium release triggers the contractile process.[1,4,6]

The metabolic characteristics of each fiber type are quite different (Table 1-2). Type 1 fibers have an abundance of mitochondria, resulting in a well-developed aerobic energy system. Concomitantly, they have ample capillaries to support the oxygen needs. Slow-twitch fibers have little stored glycogen in comparison to fast-twitch fibers. H-LDH isoenzyme dominates type 1 fibers, indicating that this fiber can utilize lactate as an energy source. Type 2b fibers have a poorly developed aerobic capacity with few mitochondria but a well-developed glycolytic capacity with ample glycogen stores. The M isoenzyme pattern of LDH is most evident in type 2b fibers; therefore, they are well suited for the generation of great amounts of force for short periods of time. The type 2a fiber is an intermediate: it has both a fairly well-developed aerobic and anaerobic capacity and abundant H and M-LDH. The extent to which type 2b fibers dominate the energy system depends on the type of training (i.e., endurance training improves the aerobic capacity while sprint training increases the anaerobic capacity).

Fiber Recruitment Pattern

During muscle contraction, type 1 fibers are recruited first. As more force or greater speed is required, type 2a and then type 2b fibers are superimposed as necessary. This is the recruitment pattern for all muscular activity.[1,8,16]

Therefore, if the exercise is relatively low in intensity and does not require a great deal of speed (e.g., jogging 12-minute mile), the type 1 fibers dominate. If the exercise requires fast movement against a great deal of resistance (e.g., sprinting or weightlifting), then not only are type 1 fibers used, type 2 fibers are called upon as necessary.

CARDIOVASCULAR SYSTEM

The components of the cardiovascular system most important during exercise are the heart and peripheral circulation. Both are controlled by the autonomic nervous system and catecholamines (epinephrine and norepinephrine), but the peripherial circulation has a local control mechanism that is extremely important during exercise (Fig. 1-2). Because the autonomics and catecholamines are intimately related, a discussion follows.

Autonomic Nervous System and Catecholamines

The sympathetic portion of the autonomic nervous system is that portion most associated with exercise.[18] It is responsible for the reaction to any stress, physical or psychological, and controls the flow of catecholamines from the adrenal medulla. This system and catecholamines, independently or simultaneously, are responsible for increasing heart rate during exercise. They also cause an increase in contractility of the heart, allowing the heart to "squeeze" out more blood with each beat. In the peripheral circulation, the sympathetics and catecholamines cause a general vasoconstriction. Mellander[19] indicated that the sympathetic nervous system is responsible for an eightfold increase in arteriolar resistance. If generalized vasoconstriction during exercise did not occur, blood pressure would decline seriously since the active muscles are vasodilating.[18] Blood pressure is the product of cardiac output and total peripheral resistance (TPR); therefore, a decrease in TPR without a concomitant increase in cardiac output results in a decrease in blood pressure (Fig. 1-2). Normally this response occurs only at the onset of exercise, since the initial increase in cardiac output is greater than the decrease in TPR.[18] Vasoconstriction also affects venous circulation, causing as much as 40 percent of the blood to be displaced into the arterial and capillary sides.[19] This displacement is important because during exercise blood flow to the muscle must be increased while blood flow to other parts of the body is maintained or decreased moderately.

Sympathetic vasoconstriction is in conflict with the needs of the working muscle, since the constriction would reduce rather than increase muscle blood flow. Therefore, two mechanisms have been postulated to cause vasodilation in the working muscle: local controls and a sympathetic dilator. Rushmer and associates[20] suggested the existence of sympathetic vasodilators in skeletal muscles, but Smith and co-workers[18] stated that no sympathetic stimulation could account for the large decrease in TPR that occurs at the local level (blood flow in the muscle increases up to 15 times during exercise). Therefore local

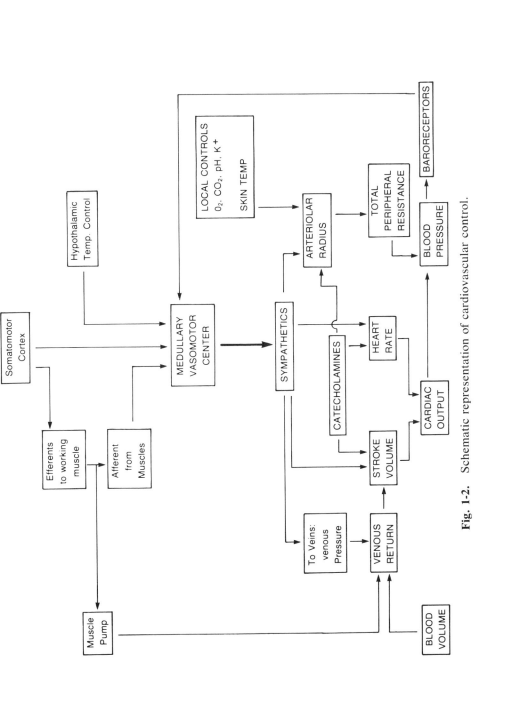

Fig. 1-2. Schematic representation of cardiovascular control.

controls are the most important influence on local blood flow during exercise. Shephard[21] noted that when the skeletal muscle sympathetics are blocked and the muscle stimulated, blood flow still dramatically increases. During exercise, this response occurs almost immediately, even when the sympathetics are blocked. The precise mechanism of the local controls is unknown but is related to local tissue hypoxia, hypercapnia, acidity, and high potassium ion concentrations.

The control of the sympathetic nervous system is speculated to be related to baroreceptor feedback, humoral feedback, cortical radiation, or afferent muscle feedback. Rushmer and associates[20] demonstrated that the somatomotor area of the cortex emits nervous impulses that travel simultaneously to both the muscles and the vasomotor areas in the medulla. Since no feedback signals are received by the central nervous system to analyze the effectiveness of the cardiovascular system in meeting the needs, this open-ended, nonfeedback mechanism has been criticized.[18] The possibility of using humoral feedback to control the cardiovascular system is very attractive. It is easy to imagine a system in which changes in the blood levels of oxygen, carbon dioxide, or another blood constituent could be monitored by a sensor and signals sent back to the vasomotor areas to affect cardiovascular functioning. Close examination of the humoral inputs has shown that changes in these occur only on the venous side; therefore, the sensor must be located there. In the past 70 years of investigation, no sensors have been found on the venous side, only on the arterial side, where blood is already normalized.

The third mechanism postulated for exercise vascular control in the working muscle involves the baroreceptors. Warner[22] noted that upon the initiation of exercise an almost immediate vasodilation occurs, lowering the total peripheral resistance. As a result, blood pressure starts to decline. The decline is sensed by the baroreceptors, which in turn activate the sympathetic nervous system, causing an increase in cardiac output and a vasoconstriction to restore blood pressure. There are serious doubts about this theory as not all studies have noted a decline in blood pressure upon the initiation of exercise.[23,24] Also, research has indicated that the baroreceptors sensitivity may diminish with training.[25]

The fourth possible mechanism of vascular control in the working muscle involves neural feedback from the exercising muscle.[26,27] When the muscle contracts, neural signals are sent back to the brain, which in turn excites the vasomotor areas. Coote and co-workers[28] and Tibes[29] demonstrated the existence of small afferent neurons that, when stimulated, affect blood pressure in direct relationship to the intensity of the stimulus. It is possible that all of these mechanisms play a role. Probably one central command from the somatomotor area of the cortex initiates the response and the baroreceptors, muscle feedback, and even humoral signals from the arterial side then act as modulators to "fine tune" the signal.

Regardless of the control mechanisms, a precise link between circulation and metabolism exists such that oxygen uptake can be calculated with the cardiac output (Q) and arterial–venous oxygen difference (a–vO$_2$):

$$VO_2 = Q \times a{-}vO_2$$

Cardiac output is the product of stroke volume and heart rate (Fig. 1–2). Heart rate is controlled by the sympathetics and catecholamines. Stroke volume is not only dependent on the sympathetics and catecholamines but, to a greater extent, on venous return.[18,30] Venous return during exercise is dependent on venous pressure and the muscle pump returning blood volume. In the normal human, cardiac output is always matched to venous return. The a–vO$_2$ difference is related to the oxygen-carrying capacity of the blood and to the tissue oxygen extraction. The oxygen-carrying capacity is based on the hemoglobin concentration with 1 g of hemoglobin transporting approximately 1.34 ml of oxygen.[1,4,6] Normal hemoglobin levels range from 12 to 15 g/100 ml blood, slightly less in girls and women than in boys and men and in trained endurance athletes. At rest, the extraction usually is about 5 ml O$_2$ per 100 ml blood. During maximal exercise the extraction can be as great as 17 ml O$_2$ per 100 ml blood.[6]

Cardiovascular Thermoregulation

A thermal load, such as occurs with prolonged exercise, places an additional stress on the cardiovascular system. Heat is removed from the body by vasodilation of the skin vessels. This change means that a portion of the blood must be redirected from the splanchnic area or muscle to the skin.[31] During mild exercise, the metabolic needs of the muscle can be maintained in spite of an increased peripheral vasodilation. During strenuous exercise, however, the metabolic needs of the muscle may be in direct conflict with the need to reduce heat stores. In this case, the blood volume being sent to the dilated skin and muscle may be so great that venous return is compromised, hence reducing cardiac output and lowering blood pressure. Normally, the body can compensate for reduced venous return by increasing heart rate, thereby maintaining cardiac output and blood pressure. Only in severe cases of heat stress is a decrease in blood pressure evident. In many cases of thermal stress the muscle blood flow is reduced and the intensity of exertion simultaneously declines.[31,32]

RESPIRATION DURING EXERCISE

The control of respiration during exercise has been an area of controversy since the beginning of the 1900s. There are two major theories, one involving humoral input, the other involving neural input. The humoral theory states that certain factors in the blood, namely oxygen, carbon dioxide, and pH, are monitored by receptors that send the information back to the respiratory control centers in the medulla which affect ventilation.[33–35] Logically, this theory makes sense because the purpose of respiration is to take up oxygen and remove CO$_2$. There are some problems with this theory. For the O$_2$, CO$_2$ or pH to be normalized, the receptor (monitor) must be located on the venous side, which is where the change occur. As with the cardiovascular system, 70 years of research have failed to produce a venous chemoreceptor. The only chemoreceptors are located on the arterial side, which contains normalized blood, or in the medulla, which monitors changes in cerebral spinal fluid (which occur slowly). Even during the most strenuous exercise, the arterial blood oxygen content does not decline significantly.[36] Therefore, arterial oxygen cannot be a stimulus. For CO_2 to stimulate respiration, the concentration must increase in the arterial blood; however, during mild to moderate exercise, arterial CO_2 remains relatively constant, and during severe exercise, CO_2 declines,[36] the opposite of what is needed to stimulate respiration. Acidity of the blood stimulates respiration. During mild and moderate exercise the pH remains fairly constant: it is not until the exercise becomes severe that the pH declines, due to lactate.[36] Therefore, pH could affect respiration only during heavy exercise and could not be considered a primary mechanism for the control of respiration.

The neural theory consists of two concepts similar to the cardiovascular control theories: a muscle afferent feedback system[26,27,37,38] and a cortical feed-forward system.[39] Kao[26,27] noted that when the hind legs of a dog are electrically stimulated, ventilation is increased. He then routed the venous circulation from the first dog (neural dog) to a second dog (humoral dog); therefore, one dog was receiving the neural stimulus only and the other the humoral stimulus. Once again, on stimulation of the hind legs of the neural dog, ventilation increased. Ventilation also increased somewhat in the humoral dog. He then added a third dog to normalize the pH in the neural dog, since hyperventilation was removing too much CO_2. When the neural dog was stimulated, the ventilation in the neural dog was noted to be significantly greater than in the humoral dog. He concluded that feedback from the exercising limbs was an important stimulus for ventilation. Tibes[29] followed up by tracing the exact neural pathways involved. Recently, Eldridge and co-workers,[39] using a decerebrated cat model, noted that when the locomotor area of the hypothalamus was electrically stimulated the cat simultaneously ran and demonstrated an increase in respiration. They then induced "fictive" locomotion (cut the nerves to and from the leg muscles and measured electrical output to ensure that the motor neurons were sending signals) and still noted an increase in ventilation without any afferent feedback. They concluded that signals are emitted from some area of the brain at or above the hypothalamus that will simultaneously cause muscle contraction and increase ventilation.

As with the cardiovascular system, the control model for respiration seems to be multiplistic in nature (Fig. 1-3). There seems to be an underlying neural signal for ventilation during exercise. All of the other inputs, afferent motor feedback, chemoreceptor, catecholamines, and temperature, act as modulators to fine tune the signal.

Respiration is a function of tidal volume and breathing rate. During exercise, the increase in respiration is a result of a change in either or both of these factors.[1,4,6] Tidal volume can increase only to approximately two-thirds of the vital capacity. Thereafter, changes in ventilation must be totally related to an increase in respiratory rate. Maximal respiration is usually reached when it is no longer possible to increase respiratory rate without decreasing tidal

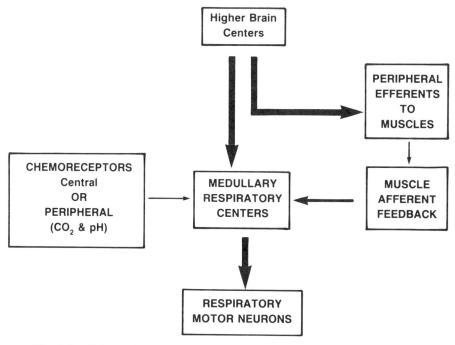

Fig. 1-3. Schematic representation of ventilatory control during exercise.

volume. Most people, with the exception of a few cyclists, have usually stopped exercising before ventilation could be considered a reason for exhaustion.

Anaerobic Threshold

Low levels of exertion result in a constant relationship between ventilation and oxygen uptake ($VE:VO_2$) of approximately 24 to 26 L of air per 1 L of oxygen uptake.[36] As the exercise becomes more strenuous and lactate is produced, the $VE:VO_2$ ratio increases. This is because the lactate is buffered, resulting in a greater CO_2 production, or is a direct effect of the lactate's lowering the blood pH.[36,40] Past research suggested that since the change in ventilation occurs at the same time blood lactate increases, this must be the point at which anaerobic metabolism becomes significant,[40,41] this point was called the "anaerobic threshold." A study by Hagberg and associates[42] has confounded the issue of the anaerobic threshold. They exercised McArdle syndrome patients, who lack some of the key enzymes of glycolysis and therefore the capacity to produce lactate. Even without the presence of anaerobiosis and significant lactate, the ventilatory threshold was evident. The significance of the anaerobic or ventilatory threshold needs clarification. The concept of the anaerobic threshold seems to be of practical significance, because many coaches and athletic trainers use this point as the level of exertion to train athletes and are successful. The onset of blood lactate and the ventilatory breakpoint are determined in a laboratory. Simultaneously, the heart rate at this point is observed. Then during workouts the heart rate is monitored to ensure that the athlete is exercising at that point of maximal aerobic involvement with minimal fatiguing lactate buildup.

OTHER SYSTEMS AND EXERCISE

In addition to the metabolic, muscular, cardiovascular, and respiratory systems, which are of primary importance during exercise, the endocrine, renal, and thermoregulatory systems play key roles. The functions of these systems are discussed below as part of the physiological events that occur as exercise processes from low to maximal intensity and exhaustion.

SEQUENCE OF INTEGRATED PHYSIOLOGICAL RESPONSES DURING EXERCISE

The exercise response can be divided into phases. Smith and co-workers[18] suggested that the cardiovascular responses to exercise can be summarized in four phases: anticipatory, initiation, adjustment, and drift. Skinner and McLellan[40] suggested that metabolically, the phase relationship to exercise is related to the intensity: low-intensity (phase 1), moderate-intensity (phase 2), and severe exercise (phase 3). I will use a combination of approaches and attempt to combine physiological events for a better appreciation of the complexity of the body's response to exercise. I will examine the anticipatory response that occurs immediately before exercise, responses that occur at the onset of exercise, the transition to steady state, severe intensity causing an acute onset of exhaustion, and prolonged exercise that leads to exhaustion (Fig. 1-4).

Anticipatory Responses

The first phase occurs just before the onset of exercise and is related to a generalized stress response brought about by psychic perception. Because the initiation of this response is psychological, the intensity of the anticipatory response depends on how stressful the individual perceives the situation. The emotional response triggers the autonomic nervous system to prepare the body: "the fight-or-flight" mechanism. The parasympathetic activity is reduced, while the sympathetic responses are enhanced. This causes heart rate to rise. Contractility of the heart increases, thus stroke volume increases. Augmentation of stroke volume and heart rate result in increased cardiac output. Guyton and co-workers[43] suggested that cardiac output can increase approximately 75 to 80 percent. The sympathetics also cause a generalized vasoconstriction. The combined effect of the vasoconstriction and increased cardiac output is to cause

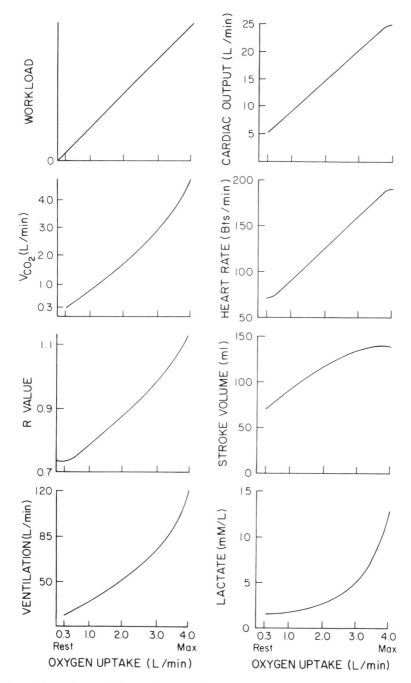

Fig. 1-4. Typical metabolic, cardiovascular, and respiratory responses to incremental exercise.

arterial blood pressure to increase. The rise in cardiac output and pressure causes a transient increase in blood flow to the muscle even though vasoconstriction occurs. The vasoconstriction also has other effects, such as reducing blood flow to the splanchnic area and kidney. Respiration begins to increase due to the sympathetics. The rise in ventilation is related to a change in tidal volume, frequency, or both. If the psychic stimulus is sufficient, the sympathetics activate the adrenal medulla, causing an outpouring of catecholamines. This secretion intensifies the sympathetic response because the catecholamines are nothing more than larger quantities of the sympathetic neurotransmitters epinephrine and norepinephrine. The epinephrine causes an activation of phosphorylase and phosphofructokinase, thus preparing glycolysis for energy production.[1,6] Lipase is activated, thus breaking down triglycerides in the adipose tissue and increasing blood lipid levels, giving energy metabolism another source of fuel. The anticipatory response may also cause ACTH to be released from the anterior pituitary, causing the release of cortisol from the adrenal cortex. The cortisol promotes the use of FFA as a source of energy.

Onset of Exercise

The second phase, onset of exercise, includes events that occur from the first movement through the first few seconds. The responses of the body during this time occur quite rapidly, with significant increases in cardiac output, ventilation, and metabolism. The primary mechanisms are neural in nature but also include humoral inputs.

Muscle contraction initiates the entire series of events. The initial contraction involves the type 1 fibers and possibly the type 2 fibers, depending on the intensity of the first contraction.[16,44] The primary fuel for the contractions at this stage is the cellular stores of ATP–CP.[1] As the ATP is reduced, ADP increases. Alteration of this ratio enhances phosphorylase and PFK activity, thus enhancing glycolysis. The aerobic pathways also are activated by the decrease in ATP. The activation of both glycolysis and oxidative phosphorylation is not completed during the onset of exercise. Muscle contraction includes not only contractions directly involved with the exercise, but abdominal contractions.[43] The net result is a compression of the capillaries and veins, which increases venous return even before changes in heart rate and stroke volume can occur. The compression caused by the abdominal muscles causes the venous reserve in the splanchnic area to be forced toward the heart. The total effect is to "prime the pump." If heart rate increased before the venous return, the amount of blood pumped by the heart would be reduced dramatically, thus compromising the blood pressure and blood flow to the muscle.

The heart rate increases within the first second. This may be accomplished initially by vagal withdrawal and then, after a short delay, by sympathetic cardio-accelerators.[45] The exact cause of the change in the autonomics is not known, but because of the speed of response it is probably neural in nature. Studies involving denervation of the heart indicate that the rate rises more slowly and that it is not until the circulating catecholamines reach the heart that a substantial increase in heart rate is evident.[46,47] The mechanism may involve a feedforward signal from the somatomotor area of the cortex or a feedback mechanism from the contracting muscle. The sympathetics also cause contractility of the heart to improve; therefore stroke volume begins to increase. The combined effect of the heart rate and stroke volume is to increase cardiac output.

The initial peripheral vascular response is vasoconstriction, but within $\frac{1}{2}$ second from the onset of exercise, total peripheral resistance begins to decline.[48,49] The decline is related to an almost instantaneous vasodilation of the working musculature. The dilation is controlled locally and may not involve a sympathetic response.[20] Ceretelli[48] demonstrated that the decline in resistance is directly related to the intensity of exercise. The vasodilation increases blood flow to the working muscle; to compensate for the dilation, skin, kidney, and intestinal blood flow is reduced.[23,50] The reduced blood flow to the intestinal system and a sympathetic-induced reduction in gastric motility in effect reduces the digestive processes. The effect of the reduced renal blood flow is to activate the renin–angiotension–aldosterone system. Sympathetic afferent arteriolar constriction reduces pressure in the Bowman's capsule of the nephron. The juxtaglomerular apparatus senses this decrease, and renin is released into the blood stream. The renin converts angiotension I (already in the blood stream) to its active form: angiotension II. Angiotension II is then transported to the adrenal cortex, where it causes the release of aldosterone, which causes the kidney to retain sodium and water. The aldosterone response is slow and not noted during the onset of exercise, but the initial renal vasoconstriction sequesters the response.[51]

The onset of exercise may cause blood pressure to increase, decrease, or not change at all.[21,26,52] Since no agreement exists as to what happens to blood pressure, a specific mechanism cannot be hypothesized. At rest, blood pressure is continuously monitored and controlled. Cardiac output and total peripheral resistance are modified as necessary to regulate blood pressure. During exercise, it seems that cardiac output and total peripheral resistance are actively controlled and that blood pressure is a passive result of their changes. If this is the case, then it is obvious how all three blood pressure responses can be reported. An increase in cardiac output greater than the decline in total peripheral resistance results in an increase in blood pressure, while a greater change in total peripheral resistance than cardiac output results in a lower blood pressure response. However, there is general agreement that within a few seconds of the onset of exercise the blood pressure rises due to an increase in cardiac output greater than the decrease in resistance.[18] This response is entirely removed when a sympathoadrenal block is administered.[47]

Ventilation increases within the first second. The increase in ventilation is related to a change in both the rate and depth; the signal is probably neural in origin.[38] The neural signal may be a feedforward signal from the motor cortex[39] or a feedback mechanism involving the contracting muscles,[26,27,52] similar to the cardiac mechanisms. Both the respiratory and circulatory changes that occur initially are not sufficient to maintain a steady state of exercise; in some cases they are greater than necessary. Therefore, further adjustments occur until the metabolic demands can be met (if possible).

The role of the sympathetic nervous system during the onset of exercise should be apparent, as evidenced by the effect on the cardiovascular, respiratory, metabolic, gastrointestinal, and renal systems. The sympathetics also cause the adrenal medulla to release catecholamines, which further intensifies the sympathetic stress response.

Adjustment Phase to Steady State

During the adjustment phase of exercise metabolic demands are balanced with cardiovascular and respiratory responses. This complex phase may be as short as 1 minute or as long as 6 minutes, depending on the intensity of exercise. The muscle fiber and energy substrate contribution to exercise is based on the demands of the activity.

Low-intensity Exercise. During low-intensity exercise, type 1 and some type 2a muscle fibers are activated.[16,44] Energy metabolism goes through a transitional phase ending in an aerobic pathway, with FFA the dominant source of energy. During the onset of exercise the dominant source of energy was cellular ATP-CP stores. As the ATP decreases and ADP increases, glycolysis and oxidative phosphorylation are stimulated. Since circulation and ventilation at this point have not increased sufficiently to meet the metabolic demand, inadequate oxygen is available to the muscle. The lack of oxygen causes the majority of pyruvic acid (being formed by glycolysis) to be converted to lactic acid. Therefore a slight buildup of acid occurs during the onset of exercise. The amount of acid buildup depends on the intensity. During low-intensity exercise, oxygen supplies are more than adequate within a few minutes. Then pyruvic acid is converted to acetyl-CoA and enters the aerobic pathway. The H-LDH in the type 1 muscle fibers converts the lactic acid back to pyruvic acid, which also enters the aerobic pathway.[44,53] In this way, the lactate produced during the first minute of exercise is metabolized. Since the stores of ATP are replenished during low-level exertion, and since citrate is available in proportionally large quantities, phosphorylase and PFK activity are suppressed.[54] Thus the substrate for energy production comes from beta oxidation (FFA).[55] Also, as exercise continues, insulin declines, activating beta oxidation.[11]

The ventilatory response during the adjustment to steady state is characterized by a slight plateau followed by a continuous rise to steady state. The mechanism for this typical response is not understood. Mahler[56] speculated that a neural drive proportional to the metabolic rate may originate in the skeletal muscle. The chemical mediator may be related to potassium being released into the extracellular spaces. Tibes and co-workers[57] monitored the time course of the change in potassium and found that it mirrors the ventilatory pattern. Wasserman and associates[34,35] also demonstrated a close relationship between CO_2 production and ventilation. The exact mechanism of feedback to the respiratory centers is not evident, but it has been speculated that the CO_2

flux to the lungs may be important. Regardless of the mechanism, ventilation during low-intensity work increases to a steady state, at which time approximately 24 to 26 L of air are ventilated for each 1 L of oxygen taken up. To reach a ventilatory steady state usually takes 3 to 6 minutes, depending on the intensity of exercise.

Concomitant with the changes in respiration and metabolism, circulatory adjustments occur. These adjustments occur fairly rapidly and attempt to match cardiac output and a–vO$_2$ difference with oxygen uptake. To increase cardiac output, both heart rate and stroke volume may increase, the change being related to the sympathetics. Rushmer et al.[20] demonstrated with dogs that the increase in cardiac output during mild exercise is more closely related to changes in heart rate than stroke volume. In contrast, Astrand and associates[58] noted that in humans, stroke volume reaches a plateau at about 40 percent of maximal oxygen uptake, suggesting that both stroke volume and heart rate changes are responsible for the increase in cardiac output. Smith et al.[18] suggested that a 50 percent increase in stroke volume may occur during moderate intensity exercise. The increase in stroke volume is related to the venous return (Frank–Starling mechanism: the heart pumps all that it receives).[30,59]

The flow of blood to the active muscle is maintained by local controls during low-intensity exercise. Smith et al.[18] stated that if at anytime the local controls cannot maintain blood flow to match the needs of the exercising muscle, afferent feedback from the muscle will increase sympathetic outflow, which will in turn increase heart rate, contractility (stroke volume), resistance to flow in nonworking muscles, venous tone, and circulatory pressure. The outcome would be to redirect more blood to the working muscle and increase cardiac output. Since the increase in cardiac output is greater than the decline in total peripheral resistance, blood pressure should increase over resting during mild exercise.

Since cardiac output is not equalibrated with metabolism during the early transition to steady state, a–vO$_2$ difference increases. Once equilibration has been obtained, the a–vO$_2$ difference decreases, but the difference is still greater than resting values.

Moderate-intensity Exercise. Moderate-intensity exercise usually results in the use of type 1, 2a, and some 2b muscle fibers.[40,44] To meet the energy demands of moderate-intensity exercise, the rate of metabolism must increase. ATP is in shorter supply, thus the ATP:ADP ratio declines and glycolysis is enhanced by activation of phosphorylase and PFK. The M-LDH isoenzyme pattern of the type 2 fibers means that more lactic acid is formed than oxidized.[53] Also, pyruvic acid is produced rapidly, fast enough that oxygen uptake cannot entirely meet the demands for conversion of pyruvate to acetyl-CoA and lactic acid is formed. During moderate-intensity exercise, lactic acid in the blood usually does not rise above 4 mmol.[40] The presence of lactic acid reduces beta oxidation to some extent[14,15]; hence, greater reliance is placed on glucose and glycogen as sources of energy. Even though there is greater reliance on carbohydrate stores and some lactate is formed, the metabolic demands can effectively be met by aerobic metabolism.

The lactic acid formed during moderate-intensity exercise causes a slight reduction in the blood pH. Also, bicarbonate buffers in the blood attempt to neutralize the acidity, forming some excess CO_2. The net effect of the acidity and CO_2 may be sufficient to cause the chemoreceptors to respond and increase ventilation. Since moderate activity changes the muscle fiber recruitment pattern, the increase in ventilation also may be related to either neural feedback from the muscles[26] or a neural feed-forward mechanism eminating from the cortex.[39] Skinner and McLellan[40] suggested that type 1 muscle may have a constant and graded neural drive. The addition of type 2 fibers may produce a different or additional neural component. Regardless of the mechanism, ventilation increases disproportionately with oxygen uptake during moderate exercise (the $VE:VO_2$ ratio increases).

During moderate-intensity exercise, cardiac output continues to rise as a result of further increases in heart rate and stroke volume. The rise in heart rate is because of the sympathetics and catecholamines, while the stroke volume change is related to improved venous return as well as the sympathetics and catecholamines. Circulatory adjustments continue to follow the pattern outlined for low-intensity exercise. Resistance to muscle blood flow continues to decline, but cardiac output increases at a greater rate than the decline in resistance, as a result of further redistribution of splanchnic blood volume.[23,50] Hence blood pressure continues to increase.

High-intensity Exercise. High-intensity exercise (above 65 percent maximal capacity) results in the recruitment of more type 2b muscle fibers. These fibers rely on glycolysis to produce energy; because of the M-LDH isoenzyme, large quantities of lactate are produced.[53] High-intensity exercise also results in an enormous output of catecholamines, which enhance glycolysis.[60,61] Blood flow to the muscle may not be able to meet the demands of aerobiosis; therefore, there is a greater reliance on anaerobiosis. Skinner and McLellan[40] also hypothesized that at about 80 percent of the muscle's maximum tension, blood flow within the active muscle begins to be occluded, also intensifying the need for anaerobiosis. Regardless of the mechanism, beta oxidation is reduced further and the use of glycogen is increased. Hjemdahl and Fredholm[62] suggested that lactate concentrations of greater than 5 mmol cause the reesterification of FFA, reducing the amount available for substrate. This is not to say that beta oxidation is totally suppressed[63] or that the activity of the oxidative pathway is reduced: actually, the aerobic pathway involving the use of glycogen and glucose are working at maximal intensity.[1,6] The anaerobic pathway (glycolysis), which is capable of producing energy faster than the aerobic pathway, acts as an additional source of energy. Only when the acid concentration from anaerobiosis reaches extremes is the aerobic activity reduced. At this time, anaerobic metabolism also may be reduced. Individuals participating in high-intensity exercise usually fatigue quite rapidly because of the production of lactic acid and the rapid utilization of the glycogen stores. There are some exceptions: some long-distance runners can exercise at 80 to 90 percent intensity for more than 2 hours.[64] This is because either they have more than 80 percent type 1 fibers or their training has improved the aerobic capacity and reduced the anaerobic capacity so that little lactate is produced until the exercise intensity is greater than 80 percent of maximal.[64]

Severe or high intensity exercise causes further divergence of ventilation and oxygen uptake. The increase in ventilation is an attempt to compensate for the further production of lactic acid and CO_2[36] or for neural input from the addition of type 2b muscle fibers. The output of catecholamines also may affect the ventilation.[1,6] This point of noticeable divergence, or break point in the VE:VO$_2$ ratio has been called the anaerobic threshold.[40,41] Normally, ventilation continues to increase until maximal oxygen uptake has been attained. Dempsey and co-workers[65] suggested that ventilation may not be a limiting factor in maximal exercise except in some extremely trained individuals or in persons with some form of respiratory dysfunction.

During severe exercise, the sympathetics and catecholamines cause the heart rate to continue to rise until maximum is attained. Stroke volume will have increased by about 100 percent over resting before maximal heart rate is achieved.[59] Thereafter, any increase in cardiac output is related to elevations in heart rate.[1,6] At maximal exertion, the cardiac output not only supplies the exercise muscular needs but also must meet the increased demands of the respiratory musculature and the thermal load, which causes the transfer of blood to the skin. In an attempt to maintain exertion, the a–vO$_2$ increases to 15 or more ml of oxygen per 100 ml of blood. Blood pressure continues to rise with exercise intensity until maximal cardiac output has been attained. Since heart rate and stroke volume can reach a maximal limit, it is apparent that the cardiovascular system is the major limiting factor in determining maximal oxygen uptake in normal individuals.[6]

Prolonged Exercise.   Prolonged exercise produces additional circulatory, metabolic, and endocrine responses not evident during short-term exercise. Circulation becomes involved with thermoregulation and fluid retention.[32] Metabolism searches for sources of energy to maintain exercise. The endocrine system assists in both of these functions.

Moderate-intensity or severe exercise, if continued long enough, result in a thermal load. The duration necessary to produce a heat response is related to the intensity of exertion, the condition of the individual, and the environmental humidity and temperature.[32] The thermal response is controlled by both the hypothalamus and local skin temperatures, with the hypothalamus having significantly more control. The initial response to a thermal load is vasodilation of the skin, an attempt to vent the heat to the surface of the body where it can be removed by radiation, convection, or evaporation. During exercise, the most effective way to dissipate heat is evaporation: approximately 75 percent of the heat loss can come from evaporation, with up to 400 kcals hour of heat being dissipated.[4,32] The sweating response is more closely related to core temperature than skin temperature,[6,32] and core temperature is dependent on exercise intensity[6,32]; therefore, there is a direct relationship between sweating and exercise intensity.

A substantial thermal load can put the body in double jeopardy. First, blood flow to the skin is increased.[31] The increased volume is first obtained from the splanchnic areas, but if this redistribution does not suffice, then blood flow to the muscle is reduced. Loss of blood flow to the working muscle increases a–vO_2 difference and could ultimately reduce the work capacity.[4,6,31] In an attempt to maintain exercise and reduce heat, more blood is in peripheral and muscular circulation, reducing venous return. The combined effect of the reduction in both total peripheral resistance (due to the dilation) and venous return is to reduce blood pressure.[31] The baroreceptors sense the change in blood pressure and elevate the heart rate and reduce the splanchnic blood flow (via sympathetics) to improve cardiac output.[31,32] If the heart rate is already maximal and splanchnic blood flow reduced maximally, then either muscle blood flow is reduced, reducing exertion, or vasoconstriction of the periphery occurs as a last resort which reduces heat loss. However, thermoregulation takes precedence over maintenance of exercise.[6] Prolonged sweating results in dehydration and a reduced blood volume. The loss of blood volume affects venous return, giving rise to a decrease in cardiac output which, in turn, decreases both skin and muscle blood flow, futher complicating thermal balance. It is clear that heat exposure during exercise should be monitored closely to avoid complications.

Osmoreceptors in the hypothalamus monitor plasma water concentrations. An increase in osmolarity (due to sweating reducing plasma water) causes transmissions to the posterior pituitary to release antidiuretic hormone (ADH),[66] which causes the kidney to retain water. A decrease in right atrial pressure (caused by a reduced venous return) also results in an increased output of ADH. In addition, fluid retention by the kidney is facilitated by the renin–angiotension–aldosterone. The reduced blood flow to the kidney produced by the vasoconstriction activates this hormonal pathway. Sweating results in a loss of sodium, which is sensed directly by the zona reticularis of the adrenal cortex and causes the release of aldosterone to facilitate renal sodium reabsorption.[6,51]

Prolonged activity results in a mobilization of greater stores of substrate within the body. The mobilization, particularly of fats, is facilitated by the endocrines (Fig. 1-5). Growth hormone increases to mobilize fats.[61,67,68] Approximately 20 minutes of exercise is necessary to elevate blood levels of growth hormone and about 1 hour is required before any effect on fat metabolism is noted[68]; therefore, for growth hormone to be beneficial the activity must be prolonged. Triggered by the release of ACTH from the pituitary, cortisol is released in response to prolonged exercise.[61,69–71] The initial signal during exercise is not known but may be related to reduced blood glucose levels or be part of the stress response. Cortisol enhances fat mobilization, giving the muscle an additional supply of substrate.

The maintenance of blood glucose levels during prolonged exercise is important, because decreased levels have been associated with fatigue.[1,6] Insulin levels are reduced during prolonged exercise as a result of both a decrease in pancreatic production (because of the sympathetics) and increased muscular uptake.[11,72] Insulin causes the cellular uptake and storage of glucose. Enhanced uptake of glucose during exercise would be beneficial, but storage of the glucose would not be. The body can compensate for the reduced insulin because blood

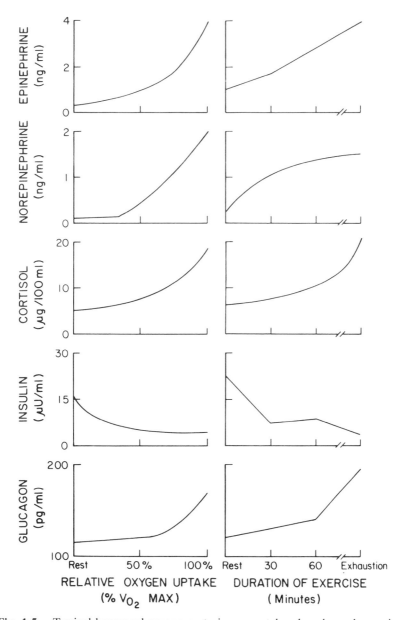

Fig. 1-5. Typical hormonal responses to incremental and prolonged exercise.

flow to the muscle is increased, bringing more glucose to the cell, and because catecholamines tend to enhance the cellular uptake of glucose.[6] Normally, blood glucose levels can be maintained for long periods of time, as long as the duration of a marathon for some individuals. But if blood glucose starts to decline, the pancreas release glucagon to stimulate liver gluconeogenesis (production of glucose from protein) to increase blood glucose levels.[73] Also, the catecholamines can stimulate the secretion of glucagon; this may occur during exercise 1 hour or longer in duration.[11,73] Since glucagon is an effervescent hormone, the effects are short-lived.

Exhaustion

The causes of exhaustion seem to be as varied as the ways an individual can exercise. Bigland–Ritchie and co-workers[74] demonstrated that the inability of the muscle to contract may originate in the central nervous system. Conversely, Stephens and Taylor[75] noted that the neuromuscular junction may be the site of exhaustion. Of course, the muscle may be the site of exhaustion; if it is, energy production or the contractile processes must be involved. For activities of short duration and severe intensity (e.g., a 100-m sprint), exhaustion may be related to depletion of the ATP–CP stores.[76,77] This activity requires a high rate of energy utilization that cannot be met by glycolysis or oxidative phosphorylation.[3] Exhaustion during activities of slightly longer duration (e.g., a 400- to 1,000-m run) may be a result of depletion of CP stores or a buildup of lactic acid, which lowers pH and reduces glycolysis.[78,79] Exhaustion during longer events (3 to 60 minutes) is not well understood, since lactate levels are not excessive and glycogen stores are not depleted. It may be related to neurological phenomenon[6] or a psychological response to the pain[80] and breathlessness.[1] Fatigue during prolonged activity (greater than 1 hour) is related to glycogen depletion,[76,79] a buildup of calcium ions in the transverse tubule system or mitochondria of the exercising muscle,[81] accumulation of ammonia (which inhibits Krebs' cycle activity [82]), dehydration,[6] or hypoglycemia.[83] Hypoglycemia (low blood glucose), which has been demonstrated to occur during marathon running, affects not only muscle metabolism but also central nervous system functioning, because the brain relies on glucose as its only source of energy.[6]

Like the causes of exhaustion, other physiological events that occur during exhaustion are not well understood. Exhaustion intensifies the stress response, particularly the adrenal catecholamine and cortisol responses (if the stress response has not been already maximally taxed).[60,61,84] If the circulation has not been maximally stressed, cardiac output increases in an attempt to supply more oxygen and metabolites to the working muscle. Respiration increases. More fats are mobilized. Blood glucagon levels may rise in response to the catecholamines in an attempt to augment depleting blood glucose levels. ADH and aldosterone levels rise in an attempt to counter any fluid and electrolyte loss. If for some reason, neurological or chemical, none of these efforts is beneficial, the stages of exhaustion ensure. Exhaustion may simply be related to the fact that muscle or brain cells have depleted their reserves and can no longer function effectively.

SUMMARY

I have reviewed the physiological responses that occur during exercise. This is not an exhaustive review of exercise physiology, but rather is intended to give insight into the intricacies of the relationships between muscle, metabolism, circulation, respiration, and endocrine systems during exercise. The mechanisms and controls of some of the responses are still speculative; much of the speculation is based on valid assumptions, and by the time of publication some of the speculation may be fact. The physiological responses, in many cases, can be modified by physical training, but it was not the purpose of this chapter to discuss any of these modifications. They are discussed in another portion of this volume.

REFERENCES

1. Brooks GA, Fahey TD: Exercise Physiology Human Bioentergetics and Its Application. Wiley, New York, 1984
2. Rafelson ME, Hayashi JA, Bezkorovainy A: Basic Biochemistry. MacMillan, New York, 1980
3. Fox EL: Sports Physiology. WB Saunders, Philadelphia, 1979
4. Astrand PO, Rodahl K: Textbook of Work Physiology. McGraw–Hill, New York, 1977
5. Gaesser GA, Brooks GA: Metabolic basis of excess post-exercise oxygen consumption: a review. Med Sci Sports Exerc 16:140, 1984
6. Lamb DR: Physiology of Exercise Responses & Adaptations. Macmillan, New York, 1984
7. Close RI: Dynamic properties of mammalian skeletal muscle. Physiol Rev 52:129, 1972
8. Saltin B: Muscle fiber recruitment and metabolism in exhaustive dynamic exercise. p. 41. In Porter R, Whelan J (eds): Human Muscle Fatigue: Physiological Mechanisms. Pitman Medical, London, 1981
9. Gollnick PD, Armstrong RB, Saubert CW et al: Enzyme activity and fiber composition of skeletal muscle of trained and untrained men. J Appl Physiol 33:312, 1972
10. Evans WJ, Fisher EC, Hoerr RA, Young VR: Protein metabolism and endurance exercise. Phys Sportsmed 11:63, 1983
11. Winder WW, Hickson RC, Hagberg JM et al: Training-induced changes in hormonal and metabolic responses to submaximal exercise. J Appl Physiol 46:766, 1979
12. Galbo H. endocrinology and metabolism in exercise. Int J Sports Med 2:203, 1981
13. Hochachka PW, Storey KB: Metabolic consequences of diving in animals and man. Science 187:613, 1975
14. Issekutz B, Shaw W, Issekutz T: Effect of lactate on FFA and glycerol turnover in resting and exercising dogs. J Appl Physiol 39:349, 1975
15. Boyd A, Giamber A, Magar M, Lebovitz H: Lactate inhibition of lipolysis in exercising man. Metabolism 23:531, 1974
16. Burke RE, Edgerton VR: Motor unit properties and selective involvement in movement. Exercise Sport Sci Rev 3:31, 1975

17. Vrbova G: Influence of activty on some characteristic properties of slow and fast twitch mammalian muscles. Exercise Sport Sci Rev 7:181, 1979

18. Smith EE, Guyton AC, Manning RD, White RJ: Integrated mechanisms of cardio-vascular response and control during exercise in the normal human. Prog Cardiovasc Dis 18:421, 1976

19. Mellander S: Comparative studies on the adrenergic neurohumoral control of resistance and capacitance blood vessels in the cat. Acta Physiol Scand, 176:suppl. 50, 1–86, 1960

20. Rushmer RF, Smith O, Franklin D: Mechanisms of cardiac control in exercise. Circ Res 7:602, 1959

21. Shephard JT: Behavior of resistance and capacitance vessels in human limbs during exercise. Circ Res 20:70, 1967

22. Warner H: The role of peripheral resistance in controlling cardiac output during exercise. Ann NY Acad Sci 115:669, 1964

23. Ekelund LG, Holmgren A: Central hemodynamics during exercise. Circ Res 20:33, 1967

24. Holmgren A: Circulatory changes during muscular work in man. Scand J Clin Lab Invest, 8:suppl. 24, 1–97, 1956

25. Stegeman J, Busert A, Brock D: Influence of fitness on the blood pressure control system in man. Aerospace Med 45:45–48, 1974

26. Kao F: the peripheral neurogenic drive: an experimental study. p.71. In Dempsey J, Reed C (eds): Muscular Exercise and the Lung. University of Wisconsin Press, Madison, 1977

27. Kao FR, Ray LH: Respiratory and circulatory responses of anesthetized dogs to induced muscular work. Am J Physiol 179:249, 1954

28. Coote JH, Hilton SM, Perez–Gonzales JE: The reflex nature of the pressor response to muscular exercise. J Physiol 215:789, 1971

29. Tibes U: Reflex inputs to the cardiovascular and respiratory centers from dynamically working canine muscles. Circ Res 41:332, 1977

30. Horwitz LD, Atkins JM, Leshin SJ: Role of the Frank–Starling mechanism during exercise. Circ Res 31:868, 1972

31. Rowell LB: Human cardiovascular adjustments to exercise and thermal stress. Physiol Rev 54:75, 1974

32. Nadel E (ed): Problems with Temperature Regulation during Exercise. Academic Press, New York, 1977

33. Byrne–Quinn E, Weil JV, Sodal IE et al: Ventilatory control in the athlete. J Appl Physiol 30:91, 1971

34. Casiburi R, Whipp BJ, Wasserman K et al: Ventilatory and gas exchange dynamics in response to sinusoidal work. J Appl Physiol 42:300, 1977

35. Wasserman DH, Whipp BJ: Coupling of ventilation to pulmonary gas exchange during nonsteady-state work in men. J Appl Physiol 54:587, 1983

36. Wasserman K, Van Kessel AL, Burton GG: Interaction of physiological mechanisms during exercise. J Appl Physiol 22:71, 1967

37. Comroe JH, Schmidt CF: Reflexes from the limbs as a factor in the hyperpnea of muscular exercise. Am J Physiol 138:536, 1943

38. DeJours P: Neurogenic factors in the control of ventilation during exercise. Circ Res 20:suppl. 1, 146, 1967

39. Eldridge FL, Milhorn DE, Waldrop TG: Exercise hyperpnea and locomotion: parallel activation from the hypothalamus. Science 211:844, 1981

40. Skinner JS, McLellan TH: The transition from aerobic to anaerobic metabolism. Res Quart Sport Exerc 51:234, 1980

41. Green HJ, Hughson RL, Orr GW, Ranney DA: Anaerobic threshold, blood lactate and muscle metabolites in progressive exercise. J Appl Physiol 54:1032, 1983
42. Hagberg JM, Coyle EF, Carroll JE et al: Exercise hyperventilation in patients with McArdle's disease. J Appl Physiol 48:540, 1980
43. Guyton AC, Douglas BH, Langston JB et al: Instantaneous increase in mean circulatory pressure and cardiac output at onset of muscular exercise. Circ Res 11:431, 1962
44. Essen B: Intramuscular substrate utilization during prolonged exercise. Ann NY Acad Sci 301:30, 1977
45. Mohrman DE, Sparks HV: Resistance and venous oxygen demands during sinusoidal exercise of dog skeletal muscle. Circ Res 33:337, 1973
46. Donald DE, Shepherd JT: Response to exercise in dogs with cardiac denervation. Am J Physiol 205:363, 1963
47. Donald DE, Ferguson DA, Milburn SE: Effect of beta-adrenergic receptor blockade on racing performance of greyhounds with normal and denervated hearts. Circ Res 22:127, 1968
48. Ceretelli P: Kinatics of adaptation of cardiac output in exercise. Proc Int Symp Phys Activ, p. 64, 1966
49. Bevegard BS, Shephard JT: Regulation of circulation during exercise in man. Physiol Rev 47:178, 1967
50. Rowell LB: Regulation of splanchnic blood flow in man. Physiologist 16:127, 1973
51. Wade CE, Claybaugh JR: Plasma renin activity, vasopressin concentration, and urinary excretory responses to exercise in man. J Appl Physiol 49:930, 1980
52. Cunningham DJC: Regulation of breathing in exercise. Circ Res 20:122, 1967
53. Sjodin B: Lactate dehydrogenase in human skeletal muscle. Acta Physiol Scand, 97:suppl. 436, 1, 1976
54. Denton R, Hughes W: Pyruvate dehydrogenase and the hormonal regulation of fat synthesis in mammalian tissues. Int J Biochem 9:545, 1978
55. Newsholme E: The regulation of intracellular and extracellular fuel supply during sustained exercise. Ann NY Acad Sci 301:81, 1977
56. Mahler MT: Neural and humoral influences on pulmonary ventilation from exercising muscle. Med Sci Sports Exercise 11:191, 1979
57. Tibes U, Hemmer B, Boning D: Heart rate and ventilation in relation to venous K^+, osmolality, pH, PCO_2, PO_2, orthophosphate, and lactate at transition from rest to exercise in athletes and non-athletes. Eur J Appl Physiol 36:127, 1977
58. Astrand PO, Cuddy TE, Saltin B et al: Cardiac output during submaximal and maximal work. J Appl Physiol 19:268, 1964
59. Braundwald E, Sonnenblick EH, Ross J: An analysis of the cardiac response to exercise. Circ Res 20:44, 1967
60. Kindermann W, Schnabel A, Schmitt WM et al: Catecholamines, growth hormone, cortisol, insulin and sex hormones in anaerobic and aerobic exercise. Eur J Appl Physiol 49:389, 1982
61. Galbo H, Holst JJ, Christensen NJ: Glucagon and plasma catecholamine responses to graded and prolonged exercise in man. J Appl Physiol 38:70, 1975
62. Hjemdahl P, Fredholm B: Comparison of the lipolytic activity of circulating and locally released noradrenaline during acidosis. Acta Physiol Scand 92:1, 1974
63. Jones NL, Heigenhauser GJF, Kuksis A et al: Fat metabolism in heavy exercise. Clin Sci 59:469, 1980
64. Foster C, Costill DL, Daniels JT, Fink WJ: Skeletal muscle enzyme activity, fiber composition and VO_2 max in relation to distance running performance. Eur J Appl Physiol 39:73, 1978

65. Dempsey JA, Vidruk EH, Mastenbrook SM: Pulmonary control systems in exercise. Fed Proc 39:1498, 1980
66. Convertino VA, Keil LC, Bernauer EM, Greenleaf JE: Plasma volume, osmolality, vasopressin, and renin activity during graded exercise in man. J Appl Physiol 50:123, 1981
67. Hartley LH: Growth hormone and catecholamine response to exercise in relation to physical training. Med Sci Sports Exercise 7:34, 1975
68. Shephard RJ, Sidney KH: Effect of physical exercise on plasma growth hormone and cortisol levels in human subjects. Exerc Sports Sci Rev 3:1, 1975
69. Farrell PA, Garthwaite TL, Gustafson AF: Plasma adrenocorticotropin and cortisol responses to submaximal and exhaustive exercise. J Appl Physiol 55:1441, 1983
70. Davis CTM, Few JD: Effects of exercise on adrenocortical function. J Appl Physiol 35:887, 1973
71. Dearman J, Francis KT: Plasma levels of catecholamines, cortisol, and beta endorphins in male athletes after running 26.2, 6, and 2 miles. J Sports Med 23:30, 1983
72. Hartley LH, Mason JW, Hogan RP et al: Multiple hormonal responses to graded exercise in relation to physical training. J Appl Physiol 33:602, 1972
73. Nilsson KD, Heding LG, Hokfelt B: The influence of short-term submaximal work on the plasma concentrations of catecholamines, pancreatic glucagon and growth hormone in man. Acta Endocrinol 79:286, 1975
74. Bigland–Ritchie B, Jones DA, Hosking GP, Edwards RHT: Central and peripheral fatigue from sustained maximal voluntary contractions of human quadriceps. Clin Sci Mol Med 54:609, 1978
75. Stephens JA, Taylor A: Fatigue of maintained voluntary muscle contraction in man. J Physiol 220:1, 1971
76. Karlsson J: Muscle ATP, CP and lactate in submaximal and maximal exercise. p. 383. In Pernow B, Saltin B (eds): Muscle Metabolism During Exercise. Plenum Press, New York, 1971
77. Karlsson J: Localized muscular fatigue: role of muscle metabolism and substrate depletion. Exerc Sports Sci Rev 7:1, 1979
78. Shalin K: Intramuscular pH and energy metabolism in skeletal muscle of man. Acta Physiol Scand 39:suppl. 455, 1, 1978
79. Saltin B, Karlsson J: Muscle glycogen utilization during work of different intensities. p. 289. In Pernow B, Saltin B (eds): Muscle Metabolism During Exercise, Plenum Press, New York, 1971
80. Elkus R, Basmajian JV: Endurance in hanging by the hands. Am J Phys Med 52:124, 1973
81. Bianchi CP, Narayan S: Muscle fatigue and the role of transverse tubules. Science 215:295, 1982
82. Mutch BJC, Bannister EW: Ammonia metabolism in exercise fatigue: a review. Med Sci Sports Exerc 15:41, 1983
83. Hultman E, Nilsson L: Liver glycogen as a glucose-supplying source during exercise. p. 179. In Keul J (ed): Limiting Factors in Physical Performance. Georg Theime Publishers, Stuttgart, 1973
84. Richter EA, Galbo H, Christensen NJ: Control of exercise induced muscular glycogenolysis by adrenal medullary hormones in rats. J Appl Physiol 50:21, 1980

2 | Physiological Effects of Training

William J. Kraemer
William L. Daniels

With the evolution of exercise science, a vast amount of information concerning the physiological effects of training has been generated. Understanding the basic training responses and adaptations of various modes of conditioning can give the clinician insights into exercise prescription. The purpose of this chapter is not to present an exhaustive review, but to provide the reader with a basic overview of the physiological effects of training.

AEROBIC TRAINING

Aerobic training results in a number of adaptations in humans. The magnitude of this response is dependent on a number of factors: the type, intensity, frequency, and duration of the training and the characteristics of the person undergoing training.

This section discusses the physiological changes associated with the adaptation to training and how the characteristics of the individual and the training itself affect this adaptation.

To determine the response to training, a measure of aerobic fitness is required. The best and most commonly measured laboratory assessment of aerobic fitness is the maximal oxygen uptake ($\dot{V}O_{2}MAX$). Astrand[1] defines $\dot{V}O_{2}MAX$ as "a measure of (1) the maximal energy output by aerobic processes,

---

* The views, opinions, and/or findings contained in this report are those of the author(s) and should not be construed as an official Department of the Army position, policy, or decision, unless so designated by other official documentation.

and (2) the functional capacity of the circulation." $\dot{V}O_2MAX$ is used to assess levels of aerobic fitness and the effects of training on aerobic fitness because it is a reliable and reproducible measure. However, to measure $\dot{V}O_2MAX$ a fair amount of expensive laboratory equipment is required. O_2 consumption can be measured while performing almost any exercise; however, for laboratory purposes the exercise is usually performed on a motor-driven treadmill or a cycle ergometer. Figure 2-1 illustrates a standard treadmill procedure for measuring $\dot{V}O_2MAX$. The values shown (approximately 45 mL/kg/min) represents a normal value for the average man 20 to 30 years of age. Oxygen consumption is usually reported as an absolute value or relative to body weight. Absolute refers simply to the amount of oxygen used each minute, for example 3.0 L/minute. For activities that require individuals to move their body weight (i.e., walking, running), values are best reported relative to body weight. In this case, someone who is walking, using 3.0 L of O_2 per minute, and has a body weight of 60 kg, would be using 50 mL/kg/min of oxygen to perform this activity. This figure is derived in the following manner:

$$\frac{3.0 \text{ L/minute}}{60 \text{ Kg}} = \frac{3,000 \text{ ml/minute}}{60 \text{ kg}} = 50 \text{ mL/kg/min}$$

Athletes generally have higher values for $\dot{V}O_2MAX$ than their sedentary counterparts.[2,3] Athletes in endurance-type sports generally have a higher $\dot{V}O_2MAX$ than other athletes.[1,2]

Numerous studies have reported increases in $\dot{V}O_2MAX$ as a result of aerobic training.[4-7] This response to training is affected by several factors. The individual's initial level of fitness is one of these factors. The effect of initial level of fitness on the response to training was classically demonstrated by Saltin and co-workers,[8] who reported that five subjects showed a 27 percent decrease in $\dot{V}O_2MAX$ as a result of 20 days of bed rest. The subjects then went on a 50-day training program. Three of these subjects had been previously sedentary and two were physically active prior to the study. The three sedentary subjects increased their $\dot{V}O_2MAX$ by 100 percent over the post-bed rest levels. The previously active subjects increased $\dot{V}O_2MAX$ by 34 percent above post-bed rest levels. When compared with initial levels of fitness, however, the sedentary and active subjects increased by 33 and 4 percent, respectively, as a result of the 50-day training program.

In another study, Daniels and co-workers[9] reported increases, no change, and decreases in the $\dot{V}O_2MAX$ values of West Point cadets during a 6-week basic training program. The response to training was dependent on the initial level of aerobic fitness; those having the lowest initial level of aerobic fitness showed an increase in $\dot{V}O_2MAX$ and those with the highest initial level of fitness showed a decrease in $\dot{V}O_2MAX$ as a result of training. This decrease appeared to be secondary to an increase in lean body weight. All three groups improved their performance in the 1.5-mile run as a result of training.

Thus the individual's initial level of fitness is an important factor to con-

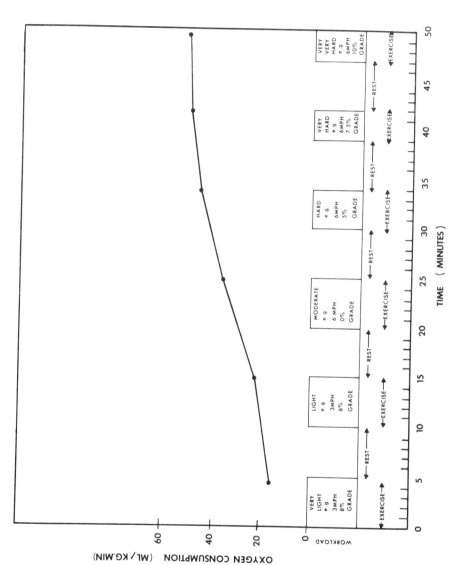

Fig. 2-1. Oxygen consumption at various exercise intensities.

sider when evaluating the response to aerobic training. Generally, the lower the initial level of fitness, the greater the percent increase in $\dot{V}O_2MAX$ as a result of training. The individual's genetic endowment may also affect this initial level of fitness and the response to training.[1]

The intensity, frequency, and duration of exercise are other factors that affect the response to training. The American College of Sports Medicine recommends a frequency of 3 to 5 days per week at an intensity between 50 and 85 percent of $\dot{V}O_2MAX$ for a duration of 15 to 60 minutes in healthy adults.[7]

Improvement in $\dot{V}O_2MAX$ in the range of 5 percent to 25 percent can be expected as a result of a moderate training program.[6,9,10] Improvements greater than this have been reported, but these are associated with low levels of initial fitness[8] or very intense and strenuous training programs.[11] The levels chosen by the American College of Sport Medicine represent those levels for intensity, duration, and frequency that will provide nonathletes with an adequate training stimulus without unnecessary risk of injury.

Studies have shown that increasing the intensity of exercise raises the dropout rate in nonathlete runners.[3] However, the importance of adequate intensity was shown by Karvonen and co-workers.[12] They showed that in two groups of young men training on a treadmill, no improvement occurred in the group that ran at a heart rate of less than 135 beats/minute, whereas significant improvement occurred in the group training at a rate greater than 153 beats/minutes.

Milesis and co-workers[13] illustrated the effect of increased duration (15, 30, and 45 minutes) of training on aerobic fitness. They found significantly greater improvement in $\dot{V}O_2MAX$ in the longest-duration group (45 minutes) compared with the 15-minute group.

Similar results were reported by Wilmore and co-workers[10] who compared 12 and 24 minutes of exercise, 3 days per week for 10 weks. While both groups showed significant increases in $\dot{V}O_2MAX$, the increase was greater in the 24-minute group.

The increase in $\dot{V}O_2MAX$ with training also has been shown to be affected by the frequency of the training. In a study that compared 2 days per week and 4 days per week of training, Pollock and co-workers[14] found twice as much of an increase in $\dot{V}O_2MAX$ (35 versus 17 percent) in the 4-day-per-week group. In another report, Pollock[3] reported increased improvement in $\dot{V}O_2MAX$ as training increased from 1 to 3 to 5 days per week. However, in this same report he also noted a marked increase in the incidence of injury as the frequency increased beyond 3 days per week and when the duration per day increased above 30 minutes.

To summarize thus far, heredity and initial level of fitness of the individual and the intensity, duration, and frequency of the training program affect the response of the individual to a training program. Because of the increased risk of injury, individuals who are just starting out are advised to begin at the lower intensity, duration, and frequency levels given in the guidelines above. It must also be remembered in the discussion to follow that these factors may modify the changes in various organ systems.

Two other factors, age and sex, should be considered. $\dot{V}O_2$MAX decreases with age in adults. This has been demonstrated by Astrand[15] and, more recently, Vogel and co-workers.[16] Vogel and associates reported a decrease in $\dot{V}O_2$MAX at an average yearly rate of 0.5 mL/kg/min in various groups of U.S. military personnel. This agrees with the average yearly decline found by Astrand and co-workers[17] in 35 women and 31 men studied in 1949 and again in 1970. Their average yearly decline was 0.438 ml/kg minute and 0.638 ml/kg minute for women and men, respectively.

Women on average, have $\dot{V}O_2$MAX values that range from 73 to 85 percent of the values of men.[9,16–19] The physiological response to training is similar in both sexes. The most noted difference is that women often show a larger increase in $\dot{V}O_2$MAX as a result of training than their male counterparts.[9,18,19] However, this is often secondary to the relatively lower initial level of fitness. The difference in $\dot{V}O_2$MAX between the sexes has been related to several factors, all of which probably have some bearing. These include a higher percentage of body fat in women, lower blood hemoglobin in women, and larger heart size and blood volumes in men.[1,16,20]

Therefore, $\dot{V}O_2$MAX is the laboratory measure most commonly used to assess aerobic fitness and the effect of an aerobic training program. The remainder of this section discusses the physiological changes that occur as a result of training and that are associated with increased aerobic fitness. The discussion is centered around the cardiovascular, cellular, and metabolic changes that occur in conjunction with an increase in $\dot{V}O_2$MAX.

For an in-depth discussion of the cardiovascular changes associated with exercise and physical training, the reader is referred to the reviews by Bevegard and Shepherd,[21] Rowell,[22] Clausen,[23] and Scheuer and Tipton.[24] $\dot{V}O_2$MAX is equivalent to the product of maximal cardiac output and arterial–venous oxygen difference, or:

$$\dot{V}O_2\text{MAX} = \text{maximal cardiac output} \times \text{a–v } O_2 \text{ difference}$$

Since cardiac output is equal to heart rate times stroke volume, oxygen consumption at any level of exercise can be calculated as:

$\dot{V}O_2$ (oxygen consumption)
$$= (\text{heart rate} \times \text{stroke volume}) \times \text{a–v } O_2 \text{ difference}$$

Aerobic training could result in a change in $\dot{V}O_2$MAX by altering any one of these variables. In reality, changes occur in all three. Heart rate is generally reduced at all submaximal exercise levels, including rest, as a result of training. Wilmore[2] stated that "resting heart rate will be reduced by 1 beat/minute for each week of participation in a moderate exercise program for previously sedentary individuals." Although this statement applies only to short-term programs, the resting heart rate is normally reduced as a result of aerobic training in all age groups.[10] Studies with rats indicate that after training the decreased heart rate may be due to increased parasympathetic activity.[24] In addition to lower resting heart rates, training results in lower heart rates at similar exercise loads.[23,24] For example, Pollock and co-workers[25] reported a decrease of 10 to 21 beats/minute in the heart rate of middle-aged men on a standard treadmill run (6.0 mph, 2.5% grade) as a result of 20 weeks of running. Yoshida and co-workers[26] reported similar findings after 8 weeks of training on a cycle ergometer. Maximal heart rate is either unchanged or slightly reduced as a result of aerobic training. This result is common in both sexes and across age groups.[9–11,19,26,27] While the decrease in heart rate at rest is due to increased parasympathetic drive, the decrease during submaximal and maximal exercise is believed to result from decreased sympathetic drive.[23,28] Cardiac output does not change substantially from the pre- to posttraining state at the same absolute workload.[1,20,28] Therefore, to maintain cardiac output in conjunction with a decreased heart rate, stroke volume has to increase. Stroke volume increases in the transition from rest to exercise in all healthy subjects up to a certain heart rate. Beyond a certain heart rate (approximately 110 beats/minute),[28] the stroke volume falls because the end diastolic volume becomes smaller. This is due to the decreased filling time available. Trained individuals have higher stroke volumes at rest and submaximal and maximal exercise.[1,26] Therefore, the same cardiac output is maintained at a reduced heart rate, making the heart more efficient. At maximal workloads, cardiac output after training is increased significantly because stroke volume is increased and heart rate is either unchanged or only slightly decreased. Rowell[22] reported that increased stroke volume accounted for approximately one half of the 15 percent increase in $\dot{V}O_2MAX$ in sedentary subjects after 3 months of training. Keul and co-workers[28] described how moderate and intensive endurance training effect stroke volume. They found that moderate training resulted in a reduction in adrenaline and noradrenaline (sympathetic drive) at the same absolute workload. This resulted in a decreased heart rate and arterial pressure. This allowed for more intensive filling of the heart and a larger end diastolic volume, as well as a decreased afterload on the heart, which allowed for a smaller end systolic volume. The overall effect is an increased stroke volume without any change in heart size. More intensive training results in an increase in heart size. Again, the increase in stroke volume is partially related due to increased end diastolic volume. Thus the pumping ability of the heart (i.e., increased stroke volume) is improved with training, but only presumptive evidence of increased contractility of cardiac muscle exists.[24]

Rowell[22] reported that approximately one half of the increase in $\dot{V}O_2MAX$ could be accounted for by increased stroke volume. The remainder of the increase was a result of an increase in the a–v O_2 difference. Adams and co-workers[29] reported similar results. This increase could be explained by two factors: first, the cardiovascular system may have become more efficient in supplying the exercising tissue with O_2; or second, the tissue may be better adapted to the use of O_2 with which it is provided.

Brooks[20] reported that after training, blood flow to active muscle is either unchanged or slightly reduced. Clausen[23] also presented evidence that during submaximal exercise, blood flow to active muscle is reduced. This, as well as other experimental findings, strongly supports the contention that trained muscles extract more oxygen from the blood. However, during maximal exercise, the blood flow to exercising muscle is also increased in the trained state.[20,23]

Scheuer and Tipton[24] suggested several possible mechanisms that might be responsible for the increased a–v O_2 difference with training. These included changes in "muscle blood flow, number of capillaries, the fiber type of muscles being recruited, alterations in concentration and activity of aerobic enzymes in cells, plus changes in the number and function of the mitochondria."

Research to date documents a number of changes in muscle cells as a result of training. These biochemical changes increase the ability of cells to perform aerobic metabolism. Thus, while no direct evidence exists conclusively to link these cellular adaptations to the increase in a–v O_2 difference, data strongly suggest that this is the case.

The remainder of this section is devoted to the cellular and metabolic changes associated with aerobic training. Reviews by Holloszy,[30] Holloszy and Booth,[31] and Howald[32] discussed the biochemical, morphological, and functional changes associated with aerobic training. Aerobic training results in a number of changes in muscle tissue itself, including increases in the density of capillaries supplying muscle fibers, increases in mitochondrial densities, changes in the substrates utilized for aerobic metabolism, increases in enzyme activities supporting oxidative reactions, and an increase in myoglobin content of muscle. Some studies also indicate that training can result in changes in muscle fiber type distribution patterns.[33,34] All of these changes assist in the maintenance of cellular homeostasis during prolonged exercise.

The number of capillaries per unit of fiber has been reported to increase with physical training and to be higher in endurance-trained athletes.[35,36] Appell[37] presented evidence to indicate that the number of capillaries does not change but that adaptations occur in capillaries as a result of training that cause them to travel a more "tortuous" route and therefore augment their cross-sectional area.

The increase in the mitochondrial densities as a result of aerobic training increases the oxidative capacity of trained muscle. Davies and co-workers[38] reported a 100 percent increase in the mitochondrial content of muscle and in the tissue oxidative capacity as a result of 10 weeks of training in rats. They reported a strong relationship between the muscle oxidative capacity and endurance performance. Holloszy and Booth[31] summarized the mitochondrial enzyme level increases that occur as a result of endurance training. These enzymes are involved in the activation and oxidation of fatty acids, in the Krebs' cycle, and in the electron transport chain. Holloszy[30] listed the increases in the specific enzymes that occur as a result of aerobic training. Training increased the levels of activity of enzymes (palmityl CoA synthetase, carnitine palmityl transferase, and palmityl CoA dehydrogenase) involved in the activation, transport, and catabolism of long-chain fatty acids. Citrate synthase, DPN-specific isocitrate dehydrogenase, and succinate dehydrogenase, all enzymes involved in the Krebs' cycle, showed a twofold increase in their level of activity as a result of endurance training. Davies and co-workers[38] reported a 108 percent increase in the mitochondrial content of succinate dehydrogenase.

Increases in the activity of components of the electron-transport chain have also been shown to occur with endurance training. Several authors[20,30,31,38] indicated that as a result of endurance training, the number and the content of muscle mitochondria are increased. The increase in activity levels, however, is an increase in total muscle activity, rather than an increase in the specific activity of the individual enzymes. Brooks and Fahey[20] presented data that show that while mitochondrial content is increased, the specific activity of the individual components of the electron transport chain is unaffected by endurance training.

According to Holloszy,[30] "when skeletal muscle adapts to endurance exercise, it becomes more like cardiac muscle in that its content of mitochondria and its capacity to generate ATP from oxidation of pyruvate and fatty acids increases."

The net result of this increase in the oxidative capacity of skeletal muscle is that submaximal exercise in the trained state causes less of an alteration in cell homeostasis. The increased capacity for fatty acid oxidation results in a slower utilization of glycogen by working muscles in the trained state. This helps prevent the depletion of glycogen, which has been demonstrated to be one of the factors limiting prolonged exercise.[39,40] The glycogen-sparing effect associated with training was demonstrated by Saltin and Karlsson.[41] They found that 6 to 8 weeks of endurance training resulted in a slower depletion of muscle glycogen for the same workload in five subjects. They also found that at the same relative percentage $\dot{V}O_2$MAX, well-trained subjects were using glycogen at a similar rate despite the fact that they were working at a higher absolute oxygen uptake. This was associated with a lower blood lactate level. One of the metabolic effects of aerobic training is a change in the workload, both absolute and percentage of $\dot{V}O_2$MAX, at which lactate begins to accumulate in the peripheral blood.[42] Gleser and Vogel[43] found that endurance time varied inversely with level of blood lactate. Blood lactate levels have been shown to be a useful measure for predicting the ability of individuals in endurance performance.

Costill and co-workers[44,45] noted that trained distance runners were capable of running at speeds much closer to maximum than untrained individuals before showing elevations in blood lactate. Since then, several investigators[46,47] have shown high correlations between some measure of blood lactate accumulation and running performance. Other investigators[48,49] have used the concept of anaerobic threshold and found strong correlations with running performance. The concept of anaerobic threshold was introduced by Wasserman and McIlroy.[50] According to their theory, at low exercise intensities, lactate is not produced by exercising muscle and blood lactate levels are the same as at rest. At some exercise intensity, blood lactate concentration begins to increase; as exercise intensifies, blood lactate progressively rises until the maximum effort is achieved. Furthermore, the theory states that these changes in blood lactate can be determined by changes in ventilatory parameters. This is based on the assumption that the rise in blood lactate concentration results in an exponential increase in ventilation as the ventilatory control mechanisms attempt to buffer lactic acid by blowing off "excess" CO_2. Lactic acid formed in muscle almost completely dissociates to hydrogen ion(H^+) and lactate. The H^+ produces CO_2 through the following reaction:

$$H^+ + \underset{\text{(bicarbonate)}}{HCO^-} = \underset{\text{(carbonic acid)}}{H_2CO_3} = \underset{\text{(carbon dioxide)}}{CO_2} + H_2O$$

They thought that the increase in blood lactate was linked to the onset of local muscle hypoxia at some workload. The word "anaerobic" was used to indicate that the supply of O_2 was not sufficient to meet all of the muscle energy demands by aerobic metabolism. Recently, there has been considerable controversy over the theory that the muscle is hypoxic and over whether ventilatory parameters are a valid indicator of lactate accumulation. The concept of anaerobic threshold was recently reviewed by a supporter[51] and an opponent[52] of the theory. Brooks[52] does not think that the accumulation of lactate is caused by muscle tissue becoming anaerobic. He presented evidence to demonstrate that sufficient O_2 is present to carry on aerobic metabolism. He believes lactate accumulation is not a result of a sudden increase in lactate production, but rather that it "is the result of (1) those processes which produce lactate and contribute to its appearance in the blood and (2) those processes which catabolize lactate after its removal from the blood." Brooks reported that in the rat, the major effect of training on lactate metabolism is an increase in lactate clearance. This has not been demonstrated in humans.

Regardless of the outcome of this controversy, lactate accumulation in blood has become a useful measure for predicting endurance performance. However, the cause and the mechanisms responsible for the accumulation and how these mechanisms are affected by training remain to be defined.

Other metabolic effects of training center around the enhancement of mobilization and utilization of free fatty acid and the glycogen sparing effect discussed earlier. An in-depth discussion of these changes is beyond the scope of this chapter; readers are referred to references 53–55. Basically, catecholamines, insulin, and glucagon are involved in regulating lipolysis, hepatic glycogenolysis, and gluconeogenesis. Galbo[53] reported that in trained and untrained subjects, the hormonal response depended on the relative rather than the absolute workload.

Other factors that can be affected favorably by aerobic training include body composition,[56] cardiovascular risk factor,[57] and psychological well-being.[58]

Summary

Aerobic training results in a number of adaptations that improve not only maximal performance but also the ability to do prolonged exercise. The amount of improvement depends on the characteristics of the individual and the training. One of the most commonly measured changes is an increase in the maximal oxygen uptake. This is associated with an increase in the maximum cardiac output. Generally, at submaximal workloads, heart rate is decreased and stroke volume is increased when compared with the untrained state. Metabolic changes include increased respiratory capacity in skeletal muscle, increased mitochondrial density and enzyme activity, and lower blood lactate levels at a given workload. Also, a shift toward the use of fatty acids for fuel occurs, which results in a glycogen-sparing effect in muscle. As a result of these adaptations, the cardiovascular system is generally considered more efficient and exercise causes less of a disturbance in the homeostasis of skeletal muscle.

RESISTANCE TRAINING

Resistance training is a popular form of conditioning in rehabilitation, fitness, and athletics. The term *strength training* was coined from the obvious objective of most resistance exercise programs. In this chapter the term *strength* refers to the muscle's ability to produce force.[59]

The physiological alterations consequent to resistance training are not only strength improvement. Furthermore, not all resistance training programs can be classified as being the same. Depending on the choices made for program variables, such as exercise, order of exercise, number of sets, load used, and duration of rest allowed, resistance training programs can be quite diverse.[60,61] The extent of physiological variation in response to changes in these program variables remains speculative but probably runs along a continuum.[62] The vast number of programs possible with simple manipulations probably helps explain why there are so many possible resistance training programs.

As a result of variations in pretraining status of subjects, program variables, and the duration of the training period, it has been difficult to make more than general observations on the apparent effects of specific resistance training programs. In the attempt to examine the physiological effects of chronic resistance training programs, cross-sectional studies of competitive lifters (olympic lifters, power lifters, and body builders) have been undertaken. Certain limitations are inherent with this type of research, including subjective groupings of various-caliber lifters for statistical analysis, lack of a universal definition for "elite" lifters by researchers, and possible augmentation of exercise stimulus with the use of anabolic steroids. Still, it appears to be our best model to examine long-term training effects.

The classic response, which has been observed in most studies examining resistance training, is the increase in muscular strength.[62-67] Most of the research over the past four decades has focused on the program variables of the number of sets and the load used and their relationship to strength gains.

It is reasonably well-established that multiple sets of an exercise is superior to single-set systems for development of maximal strength.[68,69] Most research indicates the use of three to six sets of a particular load.[62] It would appear that diminishing returns occurs after six to eight sets.[70-72] Yet it is important to remember that these observations are for relatively novice subjects who may not have been able to tolerate the greater volume (sets × repetitions × load) of exercise stress. For experienced lifters, variation in volume of training may be essential for optimal gains in strength.[73,74]

Data from research concerning the optimal load for maximal strength gains generally suggest that gains occur with the use of a five- or six-repetition maximum (RM) loading.[62,70–72,75–79] Again, this observation is inferred from subject populations who are essentially novice weight trainers, after short training programs. There is a load continuum.[60,62,63,80] Generally, heavy loads (1 to 6 RM) results in the greatest strengths gains. Use of moderate (7 to 12 RM) to light (greater than 12 RM) produces strength gains, but the magnitude of the increase is less as one moves to the lighter loads on the continuum. Data from Anderson and Kearney[81] support this concept. They demonstrated that greatest strength gains occur with the heaviest loads and diminish with lighter loads. Atha[67] suggested that minimal returns on strength occur at about 20- to 25-RM loads.

Training is typically performed with 24 to 48 hours rest between workouts.[82,83] The greatest concern is that adequate recovery is allowed between workouts. In athletes with a great deal of training background, it is not unusual for workouts to be performed 6 days per week. A recent study by Hunter[84] demonstrated 4 consecutive days of training to be superior to alternate-day workouts. This may be related to the recovery phenomenon and requires further study.

Hakkinen[85] demonstrated the importance of pretraining status as a determinant of the magnitude of strength increase. This author showed that nonathletes unaccustomed to resistance training made increases in strength to nearly twice the degree of weight-trained athletes in one half the time. This again suggests that in low-functional-capacity individuals, gains are made easily. As one gets closer to genetic potential, more work is needed to make even small improvements.

As training periods extend to longer periods of time (i.e., over a year) the type of workouts used may need to be varied.[74] This concept has been called "cycling" or "periodization" of training.[73] By changing the workout intensity (load) and volume (sets × repetitions × load) over the course of a training period, the muscle(s) apparently responds with greater maximal strength improvement. When compared with conventional resistance training programs, periodization of training, even in a short-term program, appears to be superior for development of maximal strength.[86]

The various types of strength training contraction styles (i.e., isometric, dynamic concentric/eccentric, and isokinetic) were reviewed extensively by Fleck and Schutt.[64] Each contraction style may be appropriate for different situational demands. For example, isometric programs may be appropriate in rehabilitation where pain or injury limit the range of joint motion. Dynamic programs may be more appropriate for athletes who need to train the entire joint motion maximally.[87,88] For more definitive reviews on contraction styles and terminology, the reader is referred to references 59, 62, and 63. The effects of different contraction styles of training is related to the inherent differences between them. One must be aware of the advantages and disadvantages of each style of training. Clinical decisions need to be made for each individual case based on the need, safety, range of motion of the strength gains, and effectiveness of the exercise stimulus.

Thus development of an optimal program for improvement of strength is dependent on the initial fitness level of the subject,[89] high-intensity overload of the muscle,[63] and variation in the exercise stimulus to maintain effectiveness.[73]

Cellular Changes

Strength training causes an increase in the growth of muscle.[90-92] This process, called hypertrophy, has typically been attributed to increases in the cross-sectional area of muscle fibers, the increase in the size and number of actin and myosin filaments, and the addition of sarcomeres to existing muscle fibers.[93-97] Significant controversy has surrounded the concept of hyperplasia (the increase in the number of fibers), which could account for the increased size of muscle observed following different strength training programs. Initial evidence of hyperplasia was presented in animal studies.[98,99] Over the past 5 years, examination of body builders revealed that the cross-sectional size of muscle fibers in the triceps brachii was not any different than in untrained controls.[100,101] It appears that since the arms of these athletes were significantly larger than those of controls, the adaptation may be the result of an increase in the number of fibers. A recent study of the biceps brachii of bodybuilders contradicted previous evidence in the triceps brachii; thus the issue remains equivocal.[102]

Different strength training workouts seem to result in a significantly different response when examining the capillary density of muscle. Power lifters and olympic lifters typically perform high-intensity workouts and allow for longer rest periods (2 to 5 minutes) between sets, in contrast to bodybuilders, who use moderate- to high-intensity loads, allow very little rest between sets, and probably perform more exercises. Data from bodybuilders suggest that this type of training program may induce capillary growth, whereas power and olympic lifting may reduce it.[103,104] The physiological reason for this adaptation and the exact stimulus require more definitive study. How this may relate to aerobic function or cardiovascular fitness remains speculative, but may be related to lactate clearance mechanisms.

Strength training appears to decrease the volume density of mitochondria. In a study by MacDougall and co-workers,[105] steriological analysis indicated that the mitochondrial volume density in the triceps brachii decreased following a 6-month high-intensity resistance training program. The 26 percent reduction in mitochondrial volume density seemed to indicate that heavy-resistance training programs may not be suitable for individuals concerned with aerobic performance. Yet the limited data on compatibility of aerobic metabolism and resistance training does not seem to support this fear, as no decreases in aerobic capacity have been reported.[20] More study is needed to understand the magnitude of this response in other muscles and when using other, lower-intensity resistance programs.

Nervous System

The effects of resistance training on the nervous system response is an important factor because of the functional relationship between the nerve and the muscle.[106] Using integrated electromyogram (EMG) methodologies, Moritani and DeVries[107] demonstrated that significant strength gains can take place in the absence of any significant tissue hypertrophy in the initial stages (2 to 4 weeks) of a training program. The neural component appears to be the primary mechanism underlying initial strength gains. Yet the hypertrophy component still made the largest contribution to the increased strength observed in young men following training. This was in contrast with older men, whose increased strength was explained by a greater involvement of the neural component throughout the training period.[108] It would appear that strength gains are mediated by a different neural response to training as one grows older. It has been proposed that women may utilize similar neural mechanisms to achieve strength gains.[20] The effects of resistance training in women is not significantly different from that in men except for initial upper-body strength levels and obvious hormonal differences, which may be responsible for the lack of excessive hypertrophy observed in some men.[109]

Data suggest that the nervous system plays a very large role in the possible mediation of strength gains.[110,111] This may include an improved recruitment pattern, increased synchronization, longer tonic activity, and less inhibition.[112–115] The efficacy of these mechanisms in different muscles and the responses to different styles of resistance training remains unknown. Still, it is clear that resistance training significantly alters neural function.

Bioenergetics and Enzyme Activities

Limited data suggest that strength training increases enzyme activities involved with the splitting of energy-rich phosphates, anaerobic glycolysis, and glycogenolysis, along with oxidation of carbohydrates.[1,20,32] This is associated with increases that have been demonstrated for high-energy phosphates and glycogen following training. The main energy source for high-intensity resistance training exercise is primarily anaerobic.[1] Thus it would appear that most adaptive changes are associated with the ability to support anaerobic functions.[116–118] This is an attractive hypothesis, but it has been demonstrated that aerobic enzyme markers can increase following anaerobic training. Howald[32] maintains that "the metabolic adaptations occurring in the different fiber populations are strongly related to their recruitment pattern during exercise." With recent advances in single-fiber analysis of enzyme activities, it has been shown that most vary over more than a 10-fold range, implicating a spectrum of metabolic profiles with significant overlap between fibers.[32] Thus contractile properties do not always determine metabolic capacities. A great deal of study is still needed to determine the responses to different resistance training programs.

Cardiovascular Fitness

The ability to increase aerobic fitness using a resistance training program has been of interest to both scientist and practitioner.[119] Circuit weight-training programs utilizing light loads and low rest periods between sets and exercises were the primary programs used to examine this possibility.[120–122] Gettman and Pollock,[123] examining the various studies concerning aerobic changes using circuit weight training, found only moderate increases (5 to 8 percent) in maximal oxygen consumption to occur following this style of training. A recent study by Hurly and co-workers[121] demonstrated that no significant improvement in aerobic capacity was realized when a high-intensity, single-set circuit was used. The potential lack of aerobic stimulus for this type of express circuit training was further supported in another study examining the heart rate and oxygen consumption demands.[124] The responses were well below recommended minimal aerobic training intensity levels. Only moderate gains are realized in aerobic function using resistance training, and these are highly dependent on the individual's fitness level.[125–127] It is unlikely that endurance-trained individuals would enhance aerobic fitness by using resistance training.[128]

Preventive medicine, as it relates to diet and weight-control habits, along with exercise have gained a great deal of attention over the past 10 years and have been linked to cardiovascular health. Most studies have demonstrated that resistance training can make effective changes in body composition. The typical response is an increase in lean body mass and a reduction of the fat content.[20,129] The use of more strenuous workout schedules may produce even more drastic changes, as evidenced by the low body fat percentages (8 and 13 percent) observed in male and female competitive body builders.[130–134]

Elevation of certain blood lipids has been linked to cardiovascular disease. Aerobic exercise appears to reduce those blood lipid levels and thus reduce potential cardiovascular risk.[56] Conversely, cross-sectional studies of competitive lifters have failed to demonstrate a similar response for chronic resistance training exercise: blood lipid levels were no different than those of nonathletes.[135] This seemed to implicate a less effective role for modifying blood lipids. Hurly and co-workers[136–137] demonstrated that training programs used by body builders are associated with a more favorable lipid profile than the training programs used by power lifters. This might be related to the potential higher metabolic cost of body building workouts compared with powerlifting workouts. In addition, it was shown that the use of anabolic steroids may increase the risk of coronary disease because of the adverse effects on lipid profiles. Goldburg and co-workers[138] recently demonstrated that weight training could have a favorable result on the blood lipid levels of previously sedentary men and women (mean age, 33 and 27 years, respectively). Significant reductions were observed in the absolute values of low-density lipoprotein

(LDL) cholesterol and triglycerides, along with the ratios of total cholesterol–high-density lipoprotein (HDL) cholesterol and LDL cholesterol–HDL cholesterol. Thus resistance training may be effective in reducing blood lipid levels, but not with concurrent use of anabolic steroids.

Reduction of resting blood pressure is a common response to aerobic training presumably associated with improvements in cardiovascular fitness and health.[28,57] Conversely, resistance training has never been viewed as positively affecting resting blood pressure because of the large pressor response typically elicited with lifting activities. Furthermore, much less is known about resting and exercise blood pressure responses to resistance exercise. MacDougall and co-workers[139] reported the extreme elevations in arterial blood pressure response (255/190 to 320/250) associated with the performance of a single-arm curl and a double-leg press. Fleck and Dean[140] reported extreme increases in resistance exercise arterial blood pressure, but not of the same magnitude as in the previous study. This dispariety may be a result of the elimination of the Valsalva maneuver usually associated with weight-lifting exercise. Furthermore, the level of the competitive body builder used in each study may have been different.

The relationship of the exercise response to resting blood pressure has not been fully examined. Resting blood pressure responses of competitive lifters still are not reported as being abnormal or hypertensive.[139–141] Short-term resistance training programs have not resulted in increases in resting blood pressure response. Yet Hunter and McCarthy[142] demonstrated that not all individuals can tolerate intense anaerobic training. Resting systolic blood pressures significantly increased over the course of an intense cycling and resistance training program. This response may have been related to an overtraining syndrome and lack of any periodization of training. The responses of individual subjects were variable and again pointed to the need for individual monitoring and prescription.

Hormonal Response

At present very little is known about the hormonal response to different resistance training programs. Most of the data have been generated from partial workouts or a single-exercise response. The physiological role of hormones is typically connected with metabolic responses and growth.[53,54,143]

It has been suggested that testosterone may be both related to strength and indirectly involved in the augmentation of exercise-induced hypertrophy. Few studies have examined the responses of testosterone in men and women to resistance training exercise. Weiss and co-workers[144] described testosterone responses in men and women following a four-station exercise circuit (latissimus pull down, supine bench press, arm curl, and leg press) with a 2-minute rest period between sets and exercises. Subjects exercised at 80 percent of 1 RM. Men's testosterone levels increased significantly following the circuit, and women's did not. It was concluded that men have greater absolute testosterone responses to resistance training. These results may have implications for differences observed in muscle with hypertrophy associated with chronic resistance training in men and women. Other researchers have demonstrated similar findings but have been unable to link resting testosterone levels to strength.[145,146] Skierska[146] did not report any increases in testosterone following a 30-minute weight-lifting workout in highly trained lifters but failed to report intensity levels and whether subjects were using anabolic steroids. These data also suggest that intensity plays an important role in testosterone's response to lifting exercise.

Growth hormone appears to be sensitive to intensity and frequency of lifting.[147,148] It is involved with both metabolic and growth processes.[149] Data from Vanhelder and co-workers[148] suggest that when using a single-leg press exercise, load and frequency of exercise are determining factors involved with the response of growth hormone levels. It was noted that muscle lactate and oxygen deficit may also play regulatory roles in the response of growth hormone. A considerable amount of research needs to be done to gain greater understanding of the interface between the hormonal responses and resistance training adaptations.

ANAEROBIC TRAINING

In addition to resistance training, other conditioning programs, such as sprint running or cycling, are anaerobic in nature. This type of training may have more of a direct relationship to the motor activity of some sports. The requirement for various degrees of anaerobic endurance (moderate- to high-intensity) in some sports is great.[20,150] Depending on the percentage of the maximal power output used in training, concurrent effects on aerobic metabolism are possible. This is evidenced by the associated cellular changes and increases in maximum oxygen consumption observed with interval sprint and cycling training, which are similar to the aerobic training changes. This is probably related to the number and length of exercise intervals.[151,152] Again, all effects are on a continuum, making it difficult to determine exact thresholds for these changes. Also, the genetic predisposition of the individual plays a large role in the magnitude of the training response.[1,32]

Interval sprint or cycle training typically increases maximum oxygen consumption. Fox and co-workers[153] demonstrated that low-power and high-power output interval training in men elicits similar changes in maximum oxygen consumption but that production of lactate during heavy submaximal exercise is reduced to a greater extent with a low-power program. Similar training responses have been observed in women to account for increases in maximal oxygen consumption.[154,155]

A study by Saltin[156] suggested that the magnitude of response for maximal oxygen consumption and aerobic enzyme activity is greater for endurance training than for sprint training. The spring leg demonstrated more fast twitch cross-sectional diameter increases.

Interval and sprint-type activities appear to alter enzyme activities significantly following training.[157] Roberts and co-workers[158] demonstrated increases in enzymes (phosphofructokinase, glyceraldehyde phosphate dehydrogenase, lactate dehydrogenase, and malate dehydrogenase) following 16 training sessions consisting of 200-m runs at 90 percent maximal speed. No increases were observed for succinate dehydrogenase. The improvement in anaerobic performance was linked to increases in key anaerobic enzyme activity. Green and co-workers[159] also demonstrated that changes in enzyme profiles or fiber distributions do not occur in response to a short-term stimulus period (2 consecutive days) of supramaximal exercise.

Changes in the energy substrates stored in the muscle are similar to those that occur during resistance training and depend on the aerobic component of the training program.[32] High-energy phosphates and glycogen increase. It is unlikely that triglycerides stores are utilized significantly as a result of programs with high anaerobic components.

The effects of anaerobic training remain relatively unknown and are the topic of increasing interest for scientific inquiry.

The physiological effects of training are specifically related to the exercise stimulus. The exercise stimulus results in a multivariate response. Therefore, changes typically are not observed in only one system and are not mutually exclusive. For effective exercise prescription, a solid understanding of training responses and modalities is needed.

REFERENCES

1. Astrand PO, Rodahl K: Textbook of Work Physiology. McGraw–Hill, New York, 1977
2. Wilmore JH: Acute and chronic physiological responses to exercise. In Amsterdam EA, Wilmore JH, DeMaria AN (eds): Exercise in Cardiovascular Health and Disease. Yorke Medical Books, New York, 1977
3. Pollock ML: How much exercise is enough? Phys Sportsmed, 6:50–64, 1978
4. Burke EJ: Physiological effects of similar training programs in males and females. Res Quart, 48:510–517, 1977
5. Gettman LR, Pollock ML, Durstine JL et al: Physiological response of men to 1, 3 and 5 days per week training program. Res Quart, 47:638–646, 1976
6. Pollock ML: The quantification of endurance training programs. In Wilmore JH (ed): Exercise and Sport Science Reviews. Academic Press, New York, 1973
7. American College of Sports Medicine. Position stand on the recommended quantity and quality of exercise for developing and maintaining fitness in healthy adults. Lea and Febiger, Philadelphia, 1978
8. Saltin B, Blomquist B, Mitchell JH et al: Responses to submaximal and maximal exercise after bed rest and training. Circulation, 38: suppl. 7, 1–78, 1968
9. Daniels WL, Kowal DM, Vogel JA et al: Physiological effects of a military training program on male and female cadets. Aviat Space Environ Med, 50:562–566, 1979
10. Wilmore JH, Royce J, Girandola PH et al: Physiological alterations resulting from a 10-week jogging program. Med Sci Sports, 2:7–14, 1970
11. Hickson RC, Bomze HA, Holloszy JO: Linear increase in aerobic power induced by a strenuous program of endurance exercise. J Appl Physiol, 42:372–376, 1977

12. Karvonen M, Kentala K, Mustala O: The effects of training heart rate: a longitudinal study. Ann Med Exp Biol Fenn, 35:307–315, 1957

13. Milesis CA, Pollock ML, Bah MD et al: Effects of different durations of training on cardiorespiratory function, body composition and serum lipids. Res Quart, 47:716–725, 1976

14. Pollock ML, Cureton TK, Greninger L: Effects of frequency of training on working capacity, cardiovascular function, and body composition of adult men. Med Sci Sports, 1:70–74, 1969

15. Astrand PO: Physical performance as a function of age. JAMA, 205:105–109, 1968

16. Vogel JA, Patton JF, Mello RP et al: An analysis of aerobic capacity in a large United States population. J Appl Physiol (in press)

17. Astrand I, Astrand PO, Hallback I et al: Reduction in maximal oxygen uptake with age. J Appl Physiol, 35:649–654, 1973

18. Patton JF, Daniels WL, Vogel JA: Aerobic power and body fat of men and women during Army Basic Training. Aviat Space Environ Med, 51:492–496, 1980

19. Burke EJ: Physiological effects of similar training programs in males and females. Res Quart, 48:510–517, 1977

20. Brooks GA, Fahey TD: Exercise physiology: human bioenergetics and its application. Wiley, New York, 1984

21. Bevegard BS, Shepherd JR: Regulation of the circulation during exercise in man. Physiol Rev, 47:178–213, 1967

22. Rowell LB: Human cardiovascular adjustments to exercise and thermal stress. Physiol Rev, 54:75–159, 1974

23. Clausen JP: Effect of physical training on cardiovascular adjustments to exercise in man. Physiol Rev, 57:779–815, 1977

24. Scheuer J, Tipton CM: Cardiovascular adaptations to physical training. Ann Rev Physiol, 39:221–51, 1977

25. Pollack ML, Broida J, Kendrick A et al: Effects of training two days per week at different intensities on middle-aged men. Med Sci Sports, 4:192–197, 1972

26. Yoshida T, Suda Y, Takeuchi N: Endurance training regimen based upon arterial blood lactate: effects on anaerobic threshold. Eur J Appl Physiol, 49:223–230, 1982

27. Patton JF, Vogel JA, Bedynek J et al: Response of age forty and over military personnel to an unsupervised, self-administered aerobic training program. Aviat Space Environ Med, 54:138–143, 1983

28. Keul J, Dickhuth HH, Lehmann M et al: The athlete's heart: haemodyanamics and structure. Int J Sports Med, 3:33–43, 1982

29. Adams WC, McHenry MM, Bernaouer EM: Long-term physiologic adaptations to exercise with special reference to performance and cardiorespiratory function in health and disease. In Amsterdam EA, Wilmore JH, DeMaria AN (eds): Exercise in cardiovascular health and disease. Yorke Medical Books, New York, 1977

30. Holloszy JO: Biochemical adaptations to exercise: aerobic metabolism. In Wilmore JH (ed): Exercise and Sports Sciences Review. Academic Press, New York, 1973

31. Holloszoy JO, Booth FW: Biochemical adaptations to endurance exercise in muscle. Ann Rev Physiol, 38:273–291, 1976

32. Howald H: Training-induced morphological and functional changes in skeletal muscle. Int J Sports Med, 3:1–12, 1982

33. Janssen E, Sjodin B, Tesch P: Changes in muscle fiber type distribution in man

after physical training: a sign of fiber type transformation. Acta Physiol Scand, 97:392–397, 1978

34. Tesch P, Karlsson J, Sjoin B: Muscle fiber type distribution in trained and untrained muscles of athletes. In Komi PV (ed): Exercise and Sport Biology. Human Kinetics Publishers, Champaign, Illinois, 1982

35. Anderson P, Henicksson J: Capillary supply of the quadriceps femoris muscle in man: adaptive response to exercise. J Physiol, 270:677–690, 1970

36. Brodal P, Imgger F, Hermansen L: Capillary supply of skeletal muscle fibers in untrained and endurance trained men. Am J Sports Med, 232:H705–H712, 1977

37. Appell HJ: Morphological studies on skeletal muscle capillaries under conditions of high altitude training. Int J Sports Med, 1:103–109, 1980

38. Davies KJA, Packer L, Brooks GA: Biochemical adaptation mitochondria, muscle, and whole-animal respiration to endurance training. Arch Biochem Biophys, 209:539–554, 1981

39. Holloszy JO, Rennie MJ, Hickson RC et al: Physiological consequences of the biochemical adaptations to endurance exercise. In Milvy P (ed): The marathon: physiological, medical, epidemiological and psychological studies. Ann NY Acad Sci, 301:440–450, 1977

40. Gollnick PD: Free fatty acid turnover and the availability of substraights as a limiting factor in prolonged exercise. In Milvy P (ed): The Marathon: Physiological, Medical, Epidemiological and psychological studies. Ann NY Acad Sci, 301:64–71, 1977

41. Saltin B, Karlsson J: Muscle glycogen utilization during work of different intensities. In Pernow B, Saltin B (ed): Muscle metabolism during exercise. Plenum Press, New York, 1971

42. Hermansen L, Saltin B: Blood lactate concentration during exercise at acute exposure to altitude. In Margaia R (ed): Exercise at Altitude. Excepta Medica, Amsterdam, 1967

43. Gleser MA, Vogel JA: Effects of acute alterations of VO_2max on endurance capacity of men. J Appl Physiol, 34:443–447, 1973

44. Costill DL, Thomson H, Roberts E: Fractional utilization of the aerobic capacity during distance running. Med Sci Sports, 5:248–252, 1973

45. Costill DC: Metabolic responses during distance running. J Appl Physiol, 28:251–255, 1970

46. Farrell PA, Wilmore JH, Coyle EF et al: Plasma lactate accumulation and distance running performance. Med Sci Sports, 11:338–433, 1979

47. Sjodin B, Jacobs I: Onset of blood lactate accumulation and marathon running performance. Int J Sports Med, 2:23–26, 1981

48. Kumagai S, Tanaka K, Matsura Y et al: Relationships of the anaerobic threshold, and onset of blood lactate accumulation. J Appl Physiol, 57:640–643, 1984

49. Tanaka K, Matsura Y: Marathon performance, anaerobic threshold, and onset of blood lactate accumulation. J Appl Physiol, 57:640–643, 1984

50. Wasserman K, McIlroy MB: Detecting the threshold for anaerobic metabolism in cardiac patients during exercise. Am J Cardiol, 14:844–852, 1964

51. Davis JA: Anerobic threshold: review of the concept and direction for future research. Med Sci Sports Exercise, 17:6–18, 1985

52. Brooks GA: Anaerobic threshold: review of the concept and directions for futher research. Med Sci Sports Exerc, 17:22–31, 1985

53. Galbo H: Endocrinology and metabolism in exercise. Int J Sports Med, 2:203–211, 1983

54. Galbo H: Hormonal and metabolic adaptation to exercise. Thieme–Stratton, New York, 1983
55. Winder WW: Control of hepatic glucose production during exercise. Med Sci Sports Exerc, 17:2–5 1985
56. Sharkey BJ: Physiology of Fitness. Human Kinetics Publishers, Chicago 1979
57. Bonanno JA: Coronary risk factor modification by chronic physical exercise. In Amsterdam EA, Wilmore JH, Demaria AN (eds): Exercise in Cardiovascular Health and Disease. Yorke Medical Books, New York, 1977
58. Folkins CH, Amsterdam EA: Control and modification of stress through chronic exercise. In Amsterdam EA, Wilmore JH, DeMaria AN (eds): Exercise in Cardiovascular Health and Disease. Yorke Medical Books, New York, 1977
59. Knuttgen HG: Force, work, power and exercise. Med Sci Sports, 10:226–228, 1978
60. Kraemer WJ: Exercise prescription in weight training: a needs analysis. Natl Strength Cond Assoc J, 5:64–65, 1983
61. Kraemer WJ: Exercise prescription in weight training: manipulating program variables. Natl Strength Cond Assoc J, 5:58–59, 1983
62. Atha J: Strengthening muscle. Exerc Sport Sci Rev, 9:2–73, 1981
63. McDonagh MJN, Davies CTM: Adaptive response of mammalian skeletal muscle to exercise with high loads. Eur J Appl Physiol, 52:139–155, 1984
64. Fleck SJ, Schutt RC: Types of strength training. Orthop Clin North Am, 14:449–458, 1983
65. Delorme TL: Heavy resistance exercise. Arch Phys Med, 27:607–630, 1946
66. Delorme TL: Restoration of muscle power by heavy resistance exercise. J Bone Joint Surg, 27:665–666, 1945
67. Clarke DH: Adaptations in strength and muscular endurance resulting from exercise. Exerc Sports Sci Rev, 1:73–102, 1973
68. Berger RA: Comparison of the effect of various weight training loads on strength. Res Quart, 36:141–146, 1965
69. Clarke DH, Stull AG: Endurance training as a determinant of strength and fatigability. Res Quart, 41:19–26, 1970
70. Berger RA: Effect of varied weight training programs on strength. Res Quart, 33:168–181, 1962
71. Berger RA: Optimum repetitions for the development of strength. Res Quart, 33:334–338, 1962
72. Berger RA: Comparative effects of three weight training programs. Res Quart, 34:396–398, 1963
73. Stone MH, O'Bryant H, Garhammer J et al: A theoretical model of strength training. Natl Strength Cond Assoc J, 4:36–39, 1982
74. Matveyev L: Fundametals of Sport Training. Progress Publishers, Moscow, 1981
75. Berger RA: Comparisons of the effect of various weight training loads on strength. Res Quart, 36:141–146, 1965
76. Berger RA: Effect of varied sets of static training on dynamic strength. Am Correct Ther J, 26:52–54, 1972
77. Berger RA, Hardage B: Effect of maximum loads for each of ten repetitions on strength improvement. Res Quart, 38:715–718, 1967
78. Berger RA, Harris MW: Effects of various repetitive rates in weight training on improvements in strength and endurance. J Assoc Phys Mental Rehab, 20:205–207, 1966
79. Chui E: The effect of systematic weight training on athletic power. Res Quart, 21:188–194, 1950

80. Withers RT: Effects of varied weight training load on the strength of university freshman. Res Quart 41:110–114, 1970

81. Anderson T, Kearney JT: Effects of three resistance training programs on muscular strength and absolute and relative endurance. Res Quart Exerc Sport, 51:1–7, 1982

82. O'Shea JP: Science principles and methods of strength fitness. Addison–Wesley, Reading, Massachusetts

83. Westcott WL: Strength fitness, physiological principles and training techniques. Allyn and Bacon, Boston, 1983

84. Hunter GR: Changes in body composition, body build and performance associated with different weight training frequencies in males and females. Natl Strength Cond Assoc J, 7:26–28, 1985

85. Hakkinen K: Factors influencing trainability of muscular strength during short term and prolonged training. Natl Strength Cond Assoc J, 7:32–37, 1985

86. Stowers TJ, McMillan J, Scale D et al: The short term effects of three different strength-power training methods. Natl Strength Cond Assoc J, 5:24–27, 1983

87. Noble L, McGraw LW: Comparative effects of isometric and isotonic training programs on relative load, endurance and work capacity. Res Quart, 44:96–108, 1973

88. Stone JH, Johnson RL, Carter DR: A short term comparison of two different methods of resistance training on leg strength and power. Athl Training, 14:158–160, 1979

89. Hakkinen K, Komi PV: Changes in neuromuscular performance in voluntary and reflex contractions during strength training in man. Int J Sports Med, 4:282–288, 1983

90. Ikai M, Fukunaga T: A study on training effect on strength per unit cross-sectional area of muscle by means of ultrasonic measurement. Eur J Appl Physiol, 28:173–180, 1970

91. MacDougall JD, Ward GR, Sale DG, Sutton JR: Biochemical adaptation of human skeletal muscle to heavy resistance training and immobilization. J Appl Physiol, 43:700–703, 1977

92. McDonagh MJN, Hayward CM, Davies CTM: Isometric training in human elbow flexor muscles. J Bone Joint Surg, 65:355–358, 1983

93. Goldberg AL, Etlinger JD, Goldspink DF, Jablecki C: Mechanism of work-induced hypertrophy of skeletal muscle. Med Sci Sports, 7:248–261, 1975

94. Gollnick PD, Timson BF, Moor PL, Riedy J: Muscular enlargement and number of fibers in skeletal muscles of rats. J Appl Physiol, 50:936–943, 1981

95. MacDougall JD, Elder GCB, Sale DG et al: Effects of strength training and immobilization of human fibers. Eur J Appl Physiol, 43:25–34, 1980

96. Martin RK, Albright JP, Clarke WR, Niffenegger JA: Load-carrying effects on the adult beagle tibia. Med Sci Sports Exerc, 13:343–349, 1981

97. Dons B, Bollerup K, Bonde–Paterson F, Hanckes, S: The effect of weight-lifting exercise related to muscular fiber composition and muscle cross-sectional area in humans. Eur J Appl Physiol, 40:95–106, 1979

98. Gonyea W: Role of exercise in inducing increases in skeletal muscle fiber number. J Appl Physiol, 48:421–426, 1980

99. Ho KW, Roy RR, Tweedle DC et al: Skeletal muscle fiber splitting with weight-lifting exercise in rats. Am J Anat, 157:433–440, 1980

100. MacDougall JD, Sale DG, Elder GCB, Sutton JR: Muscle ultrastructural characteristics of elite power lifters and body builders. Eur J Appl Physiol, 48:117–126, 1982

101. Tesch PA, Larson L: Muscle hypertrophy in body builders. Eur J Appl Physiol, 49:301–306, 1982
102. MacDougall JD, Sale DG, Alway SE, Sutton JR: Muscle fiber number in biceps brachii in bodybuilders and control subjects. J Appl Physiol, 57:1399–1403, 1984
103. Schantz B: Capillary supply in hypertrophied human skeletal muscle. Acta Physiol Scand, 114:635–637, 1982
104. Tesch PA, Thorsson A, Kaiser P: Muscle capillary supply and fiber type characteristics in weight and power lifters. J Appl Physiol, 56:35–38, 1984
105. MacDougall JD, Sale DG, Moroz Jr et al: Mitochondrial volume density in human skeletal muscle following heavy resistance training. Med Sci Sports, 11:164–166, 1979
106. Thortensson A, Karlsson J, Viitasalso JHT et al: Effect of strength training on EMG of human skeletal muscle. Acta Physiol Scand, 98:232–236, 1976
107. Moritani T, DeVries HA: Neural factors versus hypertrophy in the time course of muscle strength grain. Am J Phys Med, 58:115–130, 1979
108. Moritani T, DeVries HA: Potential for gross muscle hypertrophy in older men. J Gerontol, 35:672–682, 1980
109. Baechle TR: Women in resistance training. Clin Sports Med, 3:791–807, 1984
110. Edgerton VR: Neuromuscular adaptation to power and endurance work. Can J Appl Sport Sci, 1:49–58, 1976
111. Ikai M, Steinhaus AH: Some factors modifying the expression of human strength. J Appl Physiol, 16:157–163, 1961
112. Belanger A, McComas AJ: Extent of motor unit activation during effort. J Appl Physiol, 51:1131–1135, 1981
113. Kamen G, Kroll W, Zigon ST: Exercise effects upon reflex time components in weight lifters and distance runners. Med Sci Sports Exerc, 13:198–204, 1984
114. Milner–Brown HS, Stien RB, Yemin RP: The orderly recruitment of human motor units during voluntary contractions. J Physiol, 230:359–370, 1973
115. Sale DG, McDougall JD, Upton ARM, McComas AJ: Effect of strength training upon motoneuron exitability in man. Med Sci Sports Exerc, 15:57–62, 1983
116. Edgerton VR: Mammalian muscle fiber types and their adaptability. Am Zoologist, 18:113–125, 1978
117. Hakkinen K, Alen M, Komi PV: Neuromuscular, anaerobic and aerobic performance of elite power athletes. Eur J Appl Physiol, 53:97–105, 1984
118. Saltin B, Astrand PO: Maximal oxygen uptake in athletes. J Appl Physiol, 23:353–358, 1967
119. Stone MH, Wilson GD, Blessing D, Rozenek R: Cariovascular responses to short-term olympic style weight training in young men. Can J Appl Sport Sci, 8:134–139, 1983
120. Allen TE, Byrd RJ, Smith DP: Hemodynamic consequences of circuit weight training. Res Quart, 47:299–307, 1976
121. Hurley BF, Seals DR, Ehsani AA et al: Effects of high-intensity strength training on cardiovascular function. Med Sci Sports Exerc, 16:483–488, 1984
122. Wilmore JH, Parr RBG, Girandola RN et al: Physiological alterations consequent to circuit weight training. Med Sci Sports, 10:79–84, 1978
123. Gettman LR, Pollock ML: Circuit weight training: a critical review of its physiological benefits. Phys Sports Med, 9:44–60, 1981
124. Hempel LS, Wells CL: Cardiorespiratory cost of the Nautilus express circuit. Phys Sports Med, 13:82–96, 1985
125. Gettman LR, Ayres JJ: Aerobic changes through 10 weeks of slow and fast speed isokinetic training. Med Sci Sports, 10:47, 1978

126. Gettman LR, Ayres JJ, Pollock MC et al: Physiological effects on adult men of circuit strength training and jogging. Arch Phys Med Rehab, 60:115–120, 1979

127. Gettman LR, Cutler LA, Strathman T: Physiological changes after 20 weeks of isotonic isokinetic circuit training. J Sports Med Phys Fit, 20:265–274, 1980

128. Wilmore JH: Training for sport and activity the physiological bases of the conditioning process. 2nd Ed. Allyn and Bacon, Boston, 1982

129. Wilmore JH: Alterations in strength, body composition and anthropometric measurements consequent to a 10-week weight training program. Med Sci Sports, 6:133–138, 1974

130. Freedson PS, Mihevic PM, Loucks AB, Girandola RN: Physique, body composition and psychological characteristics of competitive female body builders. Phys Sports Med, 11:85–93, 1983

131. Katch VL, Katch FI, Moffet R, Gittleson M: Muscular development and lean body weight in body builders and weight lifters. Med Sci Sports Exerc, 12:340–344, 1980

132. Pipes TV: Physiological characteristics of elite body builders. Phys Sports Med, 7:262–274, 1975

133. Sprynarova S, Parizkova J: Functional capacity and body composition in top weight lifters, swimmers, runners and skiers. Int Z Ang Physiol, 29:184–194, 1971

134. Fleck SJ: Body composition of elite American athletes. Am J Sports Med, 11:398–403, 1983

135. Farrell PA, Maksucl MG, Pollock ML et al: A comparison of plasma cholesterol, triglycerides, and high density lipoprotein–cholestrol in speed skaters, weightlifters and non-athletes. Eur J Appl Physiol, 48:77–82, 1982

136. Hurley B, Seals D, Hagborg J et al: High-density lipoprotein cholesterol in body builders v powerlifters. JAMA, 252:507–513, 1984

137. Hurley B, Seals D, Ehsani A et al: Effects of high-intensity strength training on cardiovascular function. Med Sci Sports Exerc, 10:13–15, 1978

138. Goldburg L, Elliot D, Schutz R, Kloster F: Changes in lipid and lipoprotein levels after weight training. JAMA, 252:504–506, 1984

139. MacDougall JD, Tuxen D, Sale D et al: Arterial blood pressure response to heavy resistance exercise. J Appl Physiol, 58:785–790, 1985

140. Fleck SJ, Dean LS: Influence of weight training experience on blood pressure response to exercise. Med Sci Sports Exerc, 17:185, 1985

141. Longhurst JC, Kelly AR, Gonyea WJ, Mitchell JH: Echocardiographic left ventricular masses in distance runners and weight lifters. J Appl Physiol, 48:154–162, 1980

142. Hunter GR, McCarthy JP: Pressor response associated with high-intensity anaerobic training. Phys Sport Med, 11:151–162, 1983

143. Terjung R: Endocrine response to exercise. Exerc Sport Sci Rev, 7:153–180, 1979

144. Weiss L, Cureton J, Thompson F: Comparison serum testosterone and rostenodione responses to weight lifting in men and women. Eur Appl Physiol, 50: 413–419, 1983

145. Fahey T, Rolph R, Moungmee R et al: Serum testosterone body composition and strength of young adults. Med Sci Sports, 8:31–34, 1976

146. Skierska J, Ustupska J, Biczoa B, Lukaszewski J: Effect of physical exercise on plasma cortisol, testosterone, and growth hormone levels in weight lifters. Endokrynol Pol, 27:159–165, 1976

147. Lukaszewski J, Biczowa B, Bobilewicz D, et al: Effect of physical exercise on plasma cortisol and growth hormone levels in young weight lifters. Enokrynol Pol 27:149–158, 1976

148. Vahelder W, Radomsk M, Goode R: Growth hormone response during intermittent weight lifting exercise in men. Eur J Appl Physiol, 53:31–34, 1984
149. Shephard R, Sidney K: Effects of physical exercise on plasma growth hormone and cortisol levels in human subjects. Exerc Sports Sci Rev, Academic Press Inc., New York, 1975
150. Lamb D: Physiology of exercise: responses and adaptations. Macmillan, New York, 1978
151. Fox EL: Sports Physiology. WB Saunders, Philadelphia, 1979
152. Fox EL, Mathews DK: Interval Training. WB Saunders, Philadelphia, 1974
153. Fox EL, Bartels RL, Klinzing J, Ragg K: Metabolic responses to interval training programs of high and low power output. Med Sci Sports, 9:191–196, 1977
154. Weltman A, Moffatt RJ, Stamford BA: Supramaximal training in females: effects on anaerobic power outlets anaerobic capacity, and aerobic power. J Sports Sci Med, 18: 237–244, 1978
155. Lesmes GR, Fox EL, Stevens C, Otto R: Metabolic response of females to high intensity interval training of different frequencies. Med Sci Sports, 10:229–232, 1978
156. Saltin B, Nazar D, Costill L et al: The nature or the training response: peripheral and central adaptions to one legged exercise. Acta Physiol Scand, 96:298–305, 1976
157. Thorstensson A, Sjodin B, Karlsson J: Enzyme activities and muscle strength after "sprint training" in man. Acta Physiol Scand, 94:313–318, 1975
158. Roberts AD, Billeter R, Howald H: Anaerobic muscle enzyme changes after interval training. Int J Sports Med, 3:18–21, 1982
159. Green HJ, Houston ME, Thomson JA, Fraser IG: Fiber type distribution and maximal activities of enzymes involved in energy metabolism following short-term supramaximal exercise. Int J Sports Med, 5:198–201, 1984

ADDITIONAL REFERENCES

Bass A, Mackovg E, Vitek V: Activity of some enzymes of energy supplying metabolism in rat soleus after tenotomy of synergistic muscles and in contralateral control muscle. Physiol Bohemoslov, 22:613–621, 1973
Clarke DH: Correlation between the strength/mass ratio and speed of an arm movement. Res Quart, 31:570–574, 1960
Clarke DH, Herman L: Objective determination of resistance load for ten repetitions maximum for quadriceps development. Res Quart, 26:385–390, 1955
Cunningham DA, Faulkner JA: The effect of training on aerobic and anaerobic metabolism during a short exhaustive run. Med Sci Sports, 1:65–69, 1969
DeLorme TL, Ferris BG, Gallagher JR: Effect of progressive resistance exercise on muscle contraction time. Arch Phys Med, 33:86–92, 1952
DeLuca CJ, Lefever RS, McCue MP, Xenakis AP: Behavior of human motor units in different muscles during linearly varying contractions. J Physiol, 329:113–128, 1982
Hakkinen K, Alen M, Komi PV: Neuromuscular, anaerobic, and aerobic performance characteristics of elite power athletes. Eur J Appl Physiol, 53:97–105, 1984
Houston ME, Thomson JA: The response of endurance-adapted adults to intense anaerobic training. Eur J Appl Physiol, 36:207–213, 1977
Kaneshisa H, Miyashita M: Specificity of velocity in strength training. Eur J Appl Physiol 52:104–106, 1983

Knakis C, Hickson RC: Left ventricular responses to a program of lower limb strength training. Chest 78:618–621, 1980

Menapace FJ, Hammer WJ, Ritzer TF et al: Left ventricular size in competitive weight lifters: an echocardiographic study. Med Sci Sports Exerc, 14:72–75, 1982

Moffroid MT, Whipple RH: Specificity of speed of exercise. Phys Ther, 50:1692–1699, 1970

Ohtsuki T: Decrease in grip strength induced by simultaneous bilateral exertion with reference to finger strength. Ergonomics, 24:37–48, 1981

Rack DMH, Westbury DR: The effects of length and stimulus rate on isometric tension in the cat soleus muscle. J Physiol, 204:443–460, 1969

Strauss RH, Liggett MT, Lanese RR: Anabolic steroid use and perceived effects in ten weight-trained women athletes. JAMA, 253:2871–2873, 1985

Timson BF, Bowlin BK, Dudenhoeffer GA, George JB: Fiber number, area and composition of mouse soleus muscle following enlargement. J Appl Physiol, 58:619–624, 1985

Wickiewics TL, Roy RR, Powell PL et al: Muscle architecture and force–velocity relationships in humans. J Appl Physiol, 57:435–443, 1984

3 | Methods of Training

Jeffrey E. Falkel

Chapters 1 and 2 described how the body responds to exercise and the necessary changes and requirements for the body to perform physical work. This chapter is an overview of methods to train the body for different types of physical exercise and sport. The vast improvement in athletic performance and the continued upgrading of national, Olympic, and world records have been attributed, to a large extent, to more advanced and scientifically based training programs. Coaching and training techniques have come out of the "dark ages" and now incorporate highly sophisticated and well-researched methods of training. For practically every sport or athletic activity, there are probably several well-written texts dedicated to training methodology. This chapter focuses not on any single or specific training method, but on the general principles involved in training for sport, the methods of training for aerobic and anaerobic events, and methods of weight or strength training. Several excellent texts[1-9] on exercise physiology are more detailed in the area of training methods; these are good sources for additional information.

GENERAL PRINCIPLES OF PHYSICAL TRAINING

When prescribed based on knowledge of individual's medical condition, exercise is a safe and health activity. However, before beginning a training program for any type of activity or sport, the participant should be screened for any predisposing medical condition that might be aggravated by training. Many sports medicine clinics have screening protocols for orthopaedic and cardiovascular problems. The American College of Sports Medicine has published guidelines for screening.[10] Table 3-1 presents their recommendations for conditions that contraindicated participation in an exercise program.

Table 3-1. Contraindications for Exercise Testing and Exercise Training (Out-of-Hospital Setting)

1. *Contraindications*
   1. Acute myocardial infarction
   2. Unstable or at-rest angina pectoris
   3. Dangerous arrhythmias (ventricular tachycardia or any rhythm significantly compromising cardiac function)
   4. History suggesting excessive medication effects (digitalis, diuretics, psychotropic agents)
   5. Manifest circulatory insufficiency (congestive heart failure)
   6. Severe aortic stenosis
   7. Severe left ventricular outflow tract obstructive disease (IHSS)
   8. Suspected or known dissecting aneurysm
   9. Active or suspected myocarditis or cardiomyopathy (within the past year)
   10. Thrombophlebitis—known or suspected
   11. Recent embolism, systemic or pulmonary
   12. Recent or active infectious episodes (including upper respiratory infections)
   13. High dose of phenothiazine-agents
2. *Relative Contraindications**
   1. Uncontrolled or high-rate supraventricular arrhythmias
   2. Repetitive or frequent ventricular ectopic activity
   3. Untreated severe systemic or pulmonary hypertension
   4. Ventricular aneurysm
   5. Moderate aortic stenosis
   6. Severe myocardial obstructive syndromes (subvalvular, muscular or membranous obstructions)
   7. Marked cardiac enlargement
   8. Uncontrolled metabolic disease (diabetes, thyrotoxicosis, myxedema)
   9. Toxemia or complications of pregnancy

3. *Condition Requiring Special Consideration and/or Precautions*
   1. Conduction disturbances
      a. Complete atrioventricular block
      b. Left bundle branch block
      c. Wolff-Parkinson-White anomaly or syndrome
      d. Lown-Ganong-Levine syndrome
      e. Bifascicular block (with or without 1st block)
   2. Controlled arrhythmias
   3. Fixed rate pacemaker
   4. Mitral valve prolapse (click-murmur) syndrome
   5. Angina pectoris and other manifestations of coronary insufficiency
   6. Certain medications
      a. Digitalis, diuretics, psychotropic drugs
      b. Beta-blocking and drugs of related action
      c. Nitrates
      d. Antihypertensive drugs
   7. Electrolyte disturbance
   8. Clinically severe hypertension (diastolic above 110, grade III retinopathy)
   9. Cyanotic heart disease
   10. Intermittent or fixed right-to-left shunt
   11. Severe anemia (hemoglobin below 10 gm/dl)
   12. Marked obesity (20% above optimal body weight)
   13. Renal, hepatic, and other metabolic insufficiency
   14. Overt psychoneurotic disturbances requiring therapy
   15. Neuromuscular, musculoskeletal, orthopedic, or arthritic disorders which would prevent activity
   16. Moderate to severe pulmonary disease
   17. Intermittent claudication
   18. Diabetes

* In the practice of medicine the benefits of evaluation often exceed the risks for patients with these relative contraindications.

(American College of Sports Medicine: Guidelines for Graded Exercise Testing and Exercise Prescription. pp. 12–14. Lea and Febiger, Philadelphia, 1980.)

Overload Principle

Physical training produces changes in the physiological function of the various body systems. To obtain this "training effect," the exercise stress must be sufficient to overload the physiological mechanisms or to expose them to stresses that are greater than those encountered in daily activities. The overload required to bring about a training effect is related to the individual's level of fitness: the higher the athlete's conditioning level, the more overload stress is required to improve his or her condition. Once an individual achieves a given level of fitness, further improvements in fitness are possible only with increased training stimulus. If the systems are not overloaded, the physiological condition will only be maintained, not improved.

The key to the overloading principle involves the incorporation of several aspects of training: specificity of training; assessment of the level of fitness; prescription of exercise based on frequency, intensity, time of exercise, or duration; and type of exercise.

Specificity of Training. The principle of specificity is that the individual athlete must expose himself or herself to the specific demands of an event he or she is training for to obtain a maximal benefit and training effect. Although this is a common-sense principle, many training programs do not utilize it to its fullest extent; in fact, there is some evidence that participation activities that are not sport-specific may be detrimental to performance.

The body will perform as it is trained. If an activity requires a certain movement or series of events, it must be overloaded to achieve a training effect. Most sporting and athletic events involve different types of energy demands and use various energy systems.[3] Training specifically for an overload of the appropriate system should involve all aspects of the energy requirements of the sport. Table 3-2 shows the relative percentages of each energy system involved in a variety of sports. Training programs should specifically stress the various systems; percentages of training time should coincide with the percentages of the energy system used in an activity. If the sport is marathon running, for example, then the majority (95 percent) of the training should be aerobic in nature and the remainder of the training (5 percent) should be for the anaerobic lactic acid—oxygen system. For optimal conditioning and training effect, a training program must be established to address specifically the skills involved and the energy demands of the activity.

Assessment of Physical Fitness. To obtain the desired training effect, the system must be overloaded gradually, but if it is stressed too much, the system will break down rather than improve. Therefore, it is critical to know the athlete's baseline level of fitness to overload the system adequately. Physical fitness levels are assessed with various methods of exercise testing. References 12–17 are good sources for additional information on exercise testing and for specific protocols and procedures. General considerations in exercise testing follow.

1. Exercise testing should be as specific as possible. Various modalities are available to test an individual's capacity. Ergometers for walking or running (treadmill), bicycling (cycle ergometer), arm work (arm crank ergometer), rowing (rowing ergometer), swimming (tethered swimming), and skiing (skiing ergometer). Ergometers should be selected to achieve maximal specificity of training for an individual sport.

2. The protocol should be built around the athlete as he or she will be

Table 3-2. Various Sports and Activities and Their Predominant Energy Systems

Sports or Sport Activity	% Emphasis per Energy System		
	ATP–PC and LA	LA–O_2	O_2
Baseball	80	20	—
Basketball	85	15	—
Fencing	90	10	—
Field hockey	60	20	20
Football	90	10	—
Golf	95	5	—
Gymnastics	90	10	—
Ice hockey			
a. Forwards, defense	80	20	—
b. Goalie	95	5	—
Lacrosse			
a. Goalie, defense, attack men	80	20	—
b. Midfielders, man-down	60	20	20
Recreational sports	—	5	95
Rowing	20	30	50
Skiing			
a. Slalom, jumping, downhill	80	20	—
b. Cross-country	—	5	95
Soccer			
a. Goalie, wings, strikers	80	20	—
b. Halfbacks, link men	60	20	20
Softball	80	20	—
Swimming and diving			
a. 50 m freestyle, diving	98	2	—
b. 100 m, 100 yd (all strokes)	80	15	5
c. 200 m, 200 yd (all strokes)	30	65	5
d. 400 m, 440 yd, 500 yd freestyle	20	55	25
e. 1500 m, 1650 yd	10	20	70
Tennis	70	20	10
Track and field			
a. 100 m, 100 yd; 200 m, 220 yd	98	2	—
b. Field events	90	10	—
c. 400 m, 440 yd	80	15	5
d. 800 m, 880 yd	30	65	5
e. 1500 m, 1 mile	20	55	25
f. 2 miles	20	40	40
g. 3 miles, 5000 m	10	20	70
h. 6 miles (cross-country), 10,000 m	5	15	80
i. Marathon	—	5	95
Volleyball	90	10	—
Wrestling	90	10	—

(Modified from Fox EL, Mathews DK: Interval Training: Conditioning for Sport and General Fitness. p. 18. WB Saunders, Philadelphia, 1974.)

stressed during training. Each of the ergometric devices can be adjusted precisely to increase gradually the amount of energy required to continue the activity. The athlete should run, ride, row, or swim at a training pace; workloads can be increased incrementally to stress the athlete gradually.

3.   Various physiological parameters can be measured during the exercise test. Heart rate, blood pressure, and oxygen consumption ($\dot{V}O_2$) should be measured to assess the athlete's fitness level. Blood lactate oxygen saturation, cardiac output, and other physiological parameters can be monitored also if necessary.

4.   While the measurement of oxygen consumption during an exercise test is highly recommended predictive $\dot{V}O_2$ tests based on heart rate are available. The most common of these is the Astrand protocol, a submaximal 5-minute bicycle ergometer test.[1,18] For other predictive maximal tests on a treadmill (e.g., Bruce, Balke, and Naughton), the $\dot{V}O_2$ for a given workload has been predicted and the only physiologic parameter that is measured is heart rate.[16] Although these tests are better than no physical work capacity test at all, it cannot be emphasized enough that actual $\dot{V}O_2$ measurements must be taken for the most accurate evaluation.

5.   Exercise tests can be either continuous or discontinuous and modified specifically for the athlete's sport. Protocols are also regulated either submaximally or maximally. Most submaximal protocols stop the test at a predetermined end point; in maximal exercise tests, the athlete continues until he or she is unable to work any longer. In most circumstances, a maximal exercise test is recommended[15–17] because a maximal test stresses the athlete to his or her fullest capacity and allows the most accurate prescription of training stimulus to overload the capacity sufficiently without excessively stressing the system.

6.   Exercise testing, even maximal tests, are safe if conducted by trained personnel in a well-equipped laboratory. Many universities, hospitals, and sports medicine clinics offer supervised exercise testing.

Exercise Prescription.   All exercise training programs are composed of four variables: frequency, intensity, time or duration, and type of activity (FITT). Each of these variables can be manipulated to bring about a desired training response. Specific details on each variable are presented in the sections on aerobic, anaerobic, and strength training methods.

Frequency refers to the number of exercise sessions completed in a week.

Intensity refers to the percent of maximal capacity at which the athlete trains. Many exercise physiologists consider this the most important of the four variables to improve fitness.

Time or Duration refers to the length of any given training session or workout.

Type of Activity refers to the mode of activity used during training.

For a training program to be successful, the exercise must be prescribed individually for each athlete. Otherwise, compliance, injury, and overtraining can become serious problems. It is the responsibility of the sports medicine professional to gather enough information about the athlete to enable the design of a training program that best serves that athlete.

Progression

Physical training should be progressive in nature. A fine line exists between overload and overtraining; the athlete needs to know how his or her training should progress to avoid overtraining. This is particularly true for athletes who are just starting a training program. Goals should be established that are realistic and that can be met within a given time frame. Periodic assessments of fitness can be made to measure progress and determine whether the progression is appropriate or should be adjusted. Training sessions should be scheduled to alternate "hard" and "easy" workouts. Bill Bowerman, a track and field coach in Eugene, Oregon, encouraged this alternate training in not only workouts for his track athletes but also in any training program.[19] This modulation allows for a more complete recovery from the stress of exercise without the risk of overstressing.

Fun

The final consideration in training is fun: training should be enjoyable. Athletes adhere to their training methods only if they are pleasurable. In a competitive environment, the coaching staff may need to impose some training restraints on the athlete, but they must always strive to make the sport enjoyable. Likewise, individual athletes who act as their own coach should find enjoyable ways to train if they are going to continue with their training program.

AEROBIC TRAINING

Most individual activities or sports focus primarily on aerobic training, which involves stressing the energy system that enables the body to obtain as much oxygen as it is utilizing. Aerobic training serves as a base for all sports and physical activity. Adult fitness and cardiovascular and pulmonary rehabilitation programs stress aerobic training as their method of obtaining fitness. The term "aerobic training" was popularized by Kenneth Cooper in 1968, with his book, *Aerobics*.[20] Cooper's book outlined methods to overload the cardiovascular system and improve both aerobic fitness and cardiovascular condition. While *Aerobics* focused primarily on running as a mode of exercise, a more recent book by Cooper, *The Aerobic Way*,[21] demonstrates how aerobic training can be achieved through a wide variety of different types of exercise. These books outline in great detail specific aerobic training programs for specific ages and are an excellent reference for the formulation of aerobic training programs.

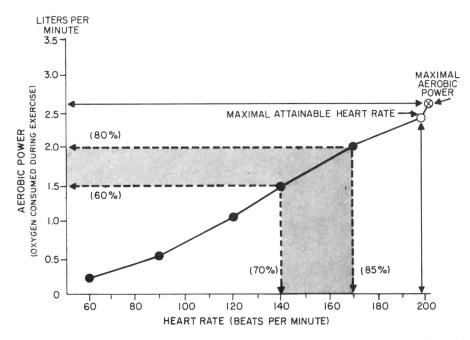

Fig. 3-1. Relationship between aerobic power and heart rate. (Zohman LR: Beyond Diet . . . Exercise Your Way to Fitness and Heart Health. p. 14. CPC International, Inc. New Jersey, 1974.)

Frequency

A great deal of research has been done to investigate the frequency of training necessary to obtain an aerobic training effect.[22-25] It has been recommended that 3 to 5 days per week of aerobic training are needed to improve fitness and that 6 days per week is the upper limit to minimize the risk of injury. Some recent studies have shown that aerobic fitness can be maintained (but not improved) by high-intensity training only 2 days per week.[26,27]

Many competitive athletes train two to three times per day, but the workouts are alternated between easy and hard, and the total time of exercise is similar. These athletes use more of an anaerobic interval training program, which is discussed later in this chapter.

Intensity

The optimal intensity for aerobic training is 60 to 80 percent of the athlete's maximal aerobic capacity, or $\dot{V}O_2MAX$. The $\dot{V}O_2$ is assessed and the standard of speed or work done at 60 and 80 percent $\dot{V}O_2MAX$ used as the training intensity range. There is a direct linear relationship between $\dot{V}O_2$ and heart rate (HR) (Fig. 3-1). An aerobic training intensity of 60 to 80 percent $\dot{V}O_2MAX$ corresponds to a heart rate of 70 to 85 percent of the maximal heart rate

(HRMAX). Because of this relationship, many aerobic training programs use an intensity of 70 to 85 percent HRMAX as a guideline.

There are both advantages and disadvantages to using heart rate to prescribe an aerobic training program. The biggest advantage is that heart rate is easy to assess: it can be monitored anywhere an artery is near a bony area (radial, carotid, brachial, etc.). Once heart rate resting (RHR) and HRMAX values are known, the Karvonen formula can be used to calculate training heart rate (THR), which is needed to obtain aerobic fitness:

$$THR_{70\%} = [(HRMAX - RHR) \times 70\%] + RHR$$

$$THR_{85\%} = [(HRMAX - RHR) \times 85\%] + RHR$$

For example, if an athlete has a HRMAX of 200 and a RHR of 50, his or her aerobic THR to obtain an intensity of 70 percent would be:

$$THR_{70\%} = [(200 - 50) \times 0.7] + 50$$
$$= [150 \times 0.7] + 50$$
$$= 155$$

His or her aerobic THR to obtain an intensity of 85 percent would be:

$$THR_{85\%} = [(200 - 50) \times 0.85] + 50$$
$$= [150 \times 0.85] + 50$$
$$= 178$$

Thus if the athlete trains at an intensity with his or her heart rate between 155 and 178, he or she will obtain an aerobic training effect.

There are several disadvantages to using heart rate as a guide to intensity. First, it makes the assumption of a HRMAX value. These values are predicted roughly from the equation

$$HRMAX = 220 - age$$

Figure 3-2 shows how both HRMAX HR and the 70 to 85 percent training zone decline with age. These values are a rough estimate of HRMAX. The only true way to assess HRMAX is during a maximal exercise test.

Another problem with using heart rate as an index of intensity is that in most individuals who are deconditioned or, conversely, extremely fit, the HR–VO_2 relationship has a different slope than that shown in Figure 3-1. Therefore the 60 to 80 percent VO_{2MAX} intensity needed for aerobic training effect will be overestimated for deconditioned persons and underestimated for extremely fit persons. Figure 3-3 demonstrates what happens to three individuals with the same THR range but different levels of aerobic capacity—only one of these

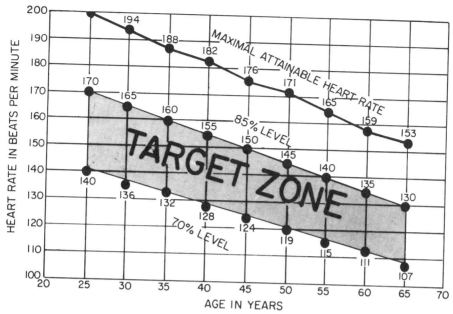

Fig. 3-2. Maximal attainable heart rate and target zone. (Zohman LR: Beyond Diet . . . Exercise Your Way to Fitness and Heart Health. p. 15. CPC International, Inc. New Jersey, 1974.)

would be getting a training effect. If oxygen consumption is not monitored and the anaerobic threshold (AT) is not measured, predicted heart rate intensities may be inaccurate. The 60 to 80 percent $\dot{V}O_2MAX$ intensity will contain the anaerobic threshold (65 to 70 percent) for healthy individuals.[29] The anaerobic threshold may be lower (40 to 50 percent) in less fit individuals, and higher (70 to 90 percent) in highly trained athletes.[28] This is a major reason for measuring $\dot{V}O_2$. Aerobic training intensities should be at or slightly below the anaerobic threshold. If the AT is not known, a THR may be too severe, causing the participant to drop out of the exercise program. If the THR is too far below the AT, the athlete will not derive the maximal training effect.

A simple rule of thumb for intensity during aerobic training is the "talk test"[19]: the intensity should not be so great that the athlete does not have enough "wind" to talk to a partner while exercising. If the athlete is unable to carry on a conversation while exercising, it probably means the intensity is too great.

Time or Duration

Most of the literature recommends a minimum of 20 to 30 minutes of exercise at the training intensity required to obtain a training effect.[10] Cooper's data indicate that a duration of longer than 45 minutes to a hour does not

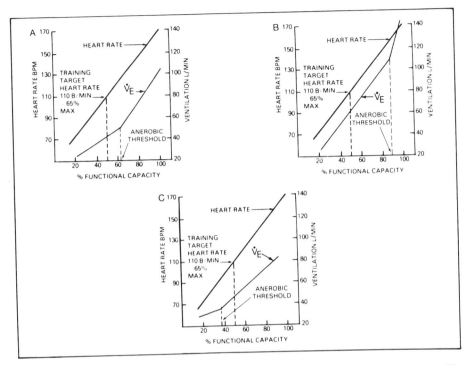

Fig. 3-3. Effect of anaerobic threshold on predicted training heart rate response. The effectiveness of a rehabilitation program may be related to the relation between the training heart rate and the anaerobic threshold. (A) Training heart rate optimal for conditioning. (B) Training heart rate too low for conditioning. (C) Training heart rate too high for accomplishment of exercise. (Wilson PK, Bell CW, Norton AC: Rehabilitation of the Heart and Lungs. p. 10. Beckman Instruments, Fullerton, CA, 1980.)

significantly improve the aerobic training effect for most activities.[21] Therefore, the recommended time for aerobic exercise is between 20 to 30 minutes and 45 minutes.

Figure 3-4 shows a typical pattern used for aerobic endurance training. The initial 5-minute warm-up is followed by the 20 to 30 minutes of stimulus at the prescribed THR. The exercise is concluded with a gradual cool-down to allow the system to return slowly to recovery levels. Recent studies show that recovery at a level below the anaerobic threshold (approximately 40 percent $\dot{V}O_2$) is more effective in removing lactic acid from the tissue than complete rest.[30] Chapter 4 details warm-up and cool-down.

The stimulus used for most aerobic endurance training methods consists of a continuous, steady-state activity (see Fig. 3-4). There are two types of continuous training: continuous-slow and continuous-fast.[4] In continuous-slow training, also called long slow distance (LSD) training, the distance covered is usually two to five times the distance traveled by the athlete in competition.[4]

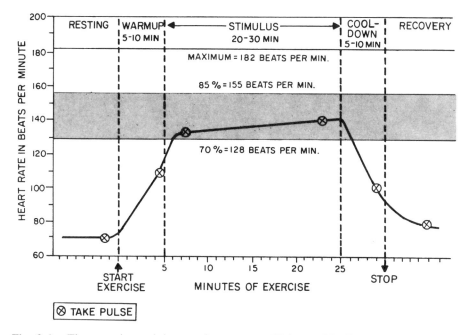

Fig. 3-4. The exercise training session pattern. (Zohman LR: Beyond Diet . . . Exercise Your Way to Fitness and Heart Health. p. 16. CPC International, Inc. New Jersey, 1974.)

In continuous-fast training, the intensity is greater but the time of the training session is shorter.

There are other forms of training, such as interval training, that will condition the aerobic system, but they are primarily anaerobic in nature. Interval training is explained in the next section.

Type or Mode of Exercise

The most common aerobic exercises are running, swimming, bicycling, rowing, cross-country skiing, and calisthenics. Most other sport activities involve more stop-and-go action. Those athletes seeking to develop a good aerobic training base will do best participating in the above activities. Cooper point-calculated more than 25 different aerobic activities that will produce an aerobic training effect.[21] With these figures, prescriptions can be formulated for a wide variety of activities to develop an aerobic training effect.

ANAEROBIC TRAINING

Most sports and athletic activities involve a substantial percentage of an anaerobic energy demand (Table 3-2). The most efficient way to train the anaerobic energy system is with interval training.

Table 3-3. Definitions of Terms Related to Interval Training

Term	Definition
Work Interval	That portion of the interval training program consisting of the work effort—e.g., a 220-yard run performed within a prescribed time.
Relief Interval	The time between work intervals in a set. The relief interval may consist of light activity such as walking (rest-relief) or mild to moderate exercise such as jogging (work-relief).
Work–Relief Ratio	The time ratio of the work and relief intervals. For example, a work-relief ratio of 1:2 means that the duration of the relief interval is twice that of the work interval.
Set	A group of work and relief intervals—e.g., six 220-yard runs (each performed within a prescribed time) separated by designated relief intervals.
Repetition	The number of work intervals per set. Six 220-yard runs would constitute 6 repetitions.
Training Time	The rate of work during the work interval—e.g., each 220-yard run might be performed in 28 seconds.
Training Distance	Distance of the work interval—e.g., 220 yards.
ITP Prescription	The specifications for the routines to be performed in an interval training workout. For example, one set from a prescription for a running program may be written as follows: Set 1 6 × 220 @ 0:28 (1:24) where: 6 = number of repetitions 220 = training distance in yards 0:28 = training time in minutes and seconds (1:24) = time of relief interval in minutes and seconds

(Fox EL: Sports Physiology. © 1979 by Saunders College Publishing/Holt, Rinehart & Winston. Reprinted by permission of CBS College Publishing.)

Interval training consists of a series of high-intensity exercise periods alternated with rest periods. The intensity of the exercise interval approximates the exercise pace used in competition. The recovery interval allows the athlete enough rest to enable him or her to complete a number of these high-quality exercise intervals.[5,11]

The design of interval training focuses around four components: the number of exercise periods; the distance of each interval; the average speed of the interval; and the length of the rest period. Table 3-3 provides definitions of the terms used with prescribe interval training.

The physiological mechanisms that enable interval training to be accomplished are discussed in previous chapters. Figure 3-5 graphically displays heart rate and oxygen consumption responses during interval training. During most of the exercise periods, the heart rate and $\dot{V}O_2$ achieve their maximal values, but during the recovery period heart rate is significantly reduced. The total work that can be accomplished with an interval training program is therefore dramatically increased (Fig. 3-6). Interval training also acts to adapt the nervous

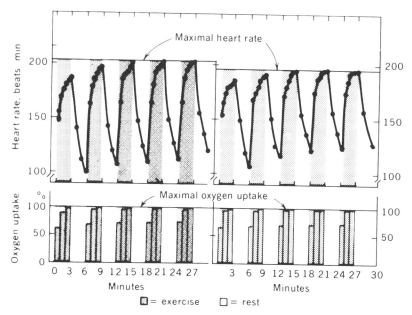

Fig. 3-5. Heart rate and oxygen uptake during interval run training. (Saltin B, Blomqvist B, Mitchell J et al: Response to submaximal and maximal exercise after bedrest and training. Circulation 38:suppl 7, 1968. By permission of the American Heart Association, Inc.)

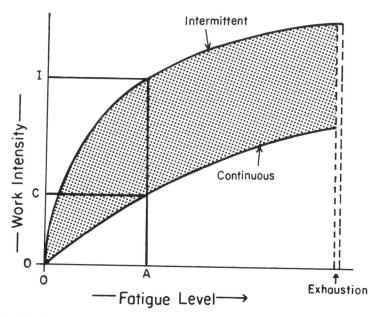

Fig. 3-6. Work performed during interval compared with continuous training. (Fox EL, Mathews DK: Interval Training: Conditioning for Sport and General Fitness. p. 25. WB Saunders, Philadelphia, 1974.)

system to the demands that are experienced in competition if the intervals are designed around the race or competition pace.[5]

Interval training can be utilized by beginning athletes or injured athletes returning to training. The short periods of exercise interspersed with rest periods allow a very deconditioned individual to improve his or her physical fitness gradually. The principles of progression for deconditioned athletes are the same as for healthy athletes. As in aerobic training, an overload of the system must occur with interval anaerobic training to produce a desired training effect. The overload can be achieved by manipulating any of the variables of interval training (Table 3-3). Longer or faster work intervals, shorter rests, and more repetitions or sets all produce an overload.

FITT Principles for Interval Training

Frequency. Because the intensity is so high with interval training, most coaches train their athletes with intervals only 2 to 3 days per week.[1,31] Track athletes and swimmers who participate in sprint events are exceptions: their training programs consist of interval training. Some coaches use the interval training as the "hard" days and alternate them with "easy" days of continuous, slow long distance aerobic training.

Intensity. The key to success with interval training is that it allows the athlete to do repeated exercise periods at or near race pace. This teaches the athlete how to sense his or her pace and regulate his or her intensity during competition. The relative intensity during the interval varies with the distance, number of repeats, and rest periods, but usually the intensity is greater than 90 percent of the athlete's $\dot{V}O_2MAX$.

Intensity is manipulated more than any other variable during interval training, depending on when in the training program the intervals are to be conducted and the athlete's response to the interval. The coach and athlete need to pay close attention to the intensity of the intervals and not allow the athlete to overtrain or break down as a result of a too-high intensity.

Time or Duration. Most research indicates equal work and recovery periods of 3 to 5 minutes,[1,4,11,31] the time of the intervals should be sport-specific. If in competition the athlete is required to extend a maximal effort for only 15 to 30 seconds, then he or she should set the interval time to simulate that pace. Athletes who must exert maximal effort for long periods should have longer intervals in training. One of the advantages of interval training is that it is sports-specific.

Type of Interval. Table 3-4 presents the definitions of various types of intervals, and Table 3-5 provides examples of selected prescriptions based on each type of interval training method.[32]

A new type of interval training, the sprint-assisted training method,[6] has been introduced in swimming and running. Essentially, this training provides a means for the athlete to go faster than he or she could normally move, either by running downhill or swimming with the assistance of an elastic recoil from tubing or with swim fins. This training produces an overload that would not

Table 3-4. Definitions of Various Training Methods and Development of the Energy Systems

Training Method	Definition	% Development		
		ATP–PC and LA	LA and O_2	O_2
Acceleration sprints	Gradual increases in running speed from jogging to striding to sprinting in 50 to 120 yd. segments	90	5	5
Continuous fast running	Long distance running (or swimming) at a fast pace	2	8	90
Continuous slow running	Long distance running (or swimming) at a slow pace	2	5	93
Hollow sprints	Two sprints interrupted by "hollow" periods of jogging or walking	85	10	5
Interval sprinting	Alternate sprints of 50 yd. and jogs of 60 yd. for distances up to 3 miles	20	10	70
Interval training	Repeated periods of work interspersed with periods of relief	10–30	30–50	20–60
Jogging	Continuous walking or running at a slow pace over a moderate distance (e.g., 2 miles)	—	—	100
Repetition running	Similar to interval training but with longer work and relief intervals	10	50	40
Speed play (fartlek)	Alternating fast and slow running over natural terrain	20	40	40
Spring training	Repeated sprints at maximal speed with complete recovery between repeats	90	6	4

(Fox EL: Physical training: methods and effects. Orthop Clin North Am, 8: 537, 1977.)

Table 3-5. Prescriptions for Various Training Methods

Training Method	Type of Athlete	Prescription
Acceleration sprints	Sprinter	Jog 50 to 120 yd., stride 50 to 120 yd., sprint 50 to 120 yd., walk 50 to 120 yd., repeat
Continuous fast running	6-miler	Run 8 to 10 miles, steady, fast pace (e.g., 10 miles/ hr.)
Continuous slow running	6-miler	Run 12 to 18 miles, steady slow pace (e.g., 8 miles/ hr.)
Hollow sprints	Sprinter	Sprint 60 yd., jog 60 yd., walk 60 yd.; repeat until fatigued
Interval sprinting	3-miler	Alternate 50 yd. sprints with 60 yd. jogs; repeat up to 3 miles
Interval training	Sprinter	Set 1 4 × 220 at 0:27 (1:21)* Set 2 8 × 110 at 0:13 (0:39) Set 3 8 × 110 at 0:13 (0:39)
	Miler	Set 1 1 × 1320 at 3:45 (1:52) Set 2 2 × 1100 at 2:58 (1:29)
Jogging	Recreational	Jog 2 miles in 14 minutes
Repetition running	Miler	Run 3 to 4 repeats of $\frac{1}{2}$ mile at a pace of 2:10 to 2:15
Speed play (fartlek)	2-miler	Jog 5 to 10 min.; run $\frac{3}{4}$ to $1\frac{1}{4}$ mi. at fast steady pace; walk 5 min.; alternate jogsprint (65–75 yd.); sprint uphill for 175–200 yd.; jog for $\frac{3}{4}$ to $1\frac{1}{4}$ mi.
Sprint training	Sprinter	Repeat full speed sprints of 60 to 70 yd. with complete recovery between repeats

* Read as follows: four 220 yd. runs at a pace of 27 seconds with one minute and 21 seconds of relief (walking) between runs.

(Fox EL: Physical training: methods and effects. Orthop Clin North Am, 8:538, 1977.)

Table 3-6. Suggested Sprint and Endurance Training Methods for Various Sports and Sports Activities

Sport or Sport Activity	Acceleration sprints	Continuous fast running	Continuous slow running	Hollow sprints	Interval sprinting	Interval training	Jogging	Repetition running	Speed play (fartlek)	Sprint training
Baseball				✓		✓				✓
Basketball				✓		✓				✓
Fencing	✓			✓		✓				✓
Field Hockey						✓				
Football	✓			✓		✓				✓
Golf	✓									✓
Gymnastics	✓			✓		✓				✓
Ice Hockey*										
Forwards, defense				✓		✓				
Goalie	✓					✓				✓
Lacrosse										
Goalie, defense, attack men				✓		✓				
Midfielders, man-down						✓				
Recreational Sports			✓			✓	✓			
Rowing*						✓		✓	✓	
Skiing*										
Slalom, jumping, downhill				✓		✓				
Cross-country		✓	✓							
Soccer										
Goalie, wings, strikers				✓		✓				
Halfbacks, link men						✓				
Softball				✓		✓				✓
Swimming and Diving*										
50 m freestyle, diving	✓									✓
100 m, 100 yd (all strokes)				✓		✓				
200 m, 220 yd (all strokes)						✓				
400 m, 440 yd freestyle						✓		✓	✓	
1500 m, 1650 yd freestyle					✓	✓				
Tennis						✓				
Track and Field										
100 m, 100 yd	✓									✓
200 m, 200 yd	✓			✓		✓				✓
Field events	✓			✓		✓				✓
400 m, 440 yd				✓		✓				
800 m, 880 yd						✓				
1500 m, 1 mile						✓		✓	✓	
2 miles						✓		✓	✓	
3 miles 5000 m					✓	✓				
6 miles, 10,000 m		✓			✓	✓				
Marathon		✓	✓							
Volleyball	✓			✓		✓				✓
Wrestling	✓			✓		✓				✓

* Rather than running, the mode of exercise during the training sessions should be that used in the sport.

(Fox EL: Sports Physiology. © 1979 by Saunders College Publishing/Holt, Rinehart & Winston. Reprinted by permission of CBS College Publishing.)

normally be provided. The additional speed allows more muscle fibers to be recruited to complete the movement,[6] so the athlete can increase the force he or she applies. More research is needed on sprint-assisted training, but it seems to hold great potential for improving performance.

Table 3-6 presents suggested types of intervals for a wide variety of sports and athletic activities. Most athletes utilize interval training as part, if not all, of their training regime and it will improve aerobic power somewhat, but it is still really the only method to improve anaerobic power.

YEAR-ROUND TRAINING

In aerobic and anaerobic training, recreational athletes or athletes not involved in competitive events may not have periods when they alter their daily training effect, except for variety. Competitive athletes, however, have three phases of training that involve different types of activities: preseason, in-season, and off-season. Pre-season training, in the 8 to 10 weeks before competition, is designed to stress the system maximally and to develop a solid foundation from which to build. During in-season training, during the competition period, quality of training is more important than quantity. Actual competitive situations, drills, scrimmages, and time trials are stressed to sharpen skills and abilities. The off-season period often is the longest, and the success of the competitive season may be determined by how fit the athlete stays during the off-season. Off-season activity should be enjoyable and not necessarily as stressful and can include recreational activities not normally done during the competitive season that can help to maintain aerobic condition. The off-season is also the best time to begin a weight-training program.

DETRAINING

The final consideration in aerobic and anaerobic training is detraining. When healthy people are confined to bed for as little as 7 days,[33] 15 days,[34] or 21 days,[35] significant reduction in maximal oxygen uptake and many other physiological consequences result. The period of retraining required to achieve pre-bedrest values is longer than the period of bedrest.[34,36] When an athlete is forced to detrain for even short perids of time, it takes careful coaching and rehabilitation to progress back to the same level of fitness. An individual who is severely deconditioned and unhealthy at the outset must progress even more slowly.

WEIGHT TRAINING

Today's athlete is bigger and stronger than ever before. Much of this increase in size is because of the number of athletes involved in weight training. Many of the general principles of training already discussed apply equally to weight training.

Overload

For a muscle to gain strength, it must be overloaded. In addition, the athlete must perform the strengthening exercises with near-maximal or maximal resistance to achieve the optimal gain in strength.[5,37]

Specificity

A muscle will perform only as it is trained; thus weight training exercises can and must be designed to mimic as closely as possible the kinds of activities that the athlete performs in his or her sport. Weight training can be a tremendous supplement to an athlete's ability if the exercises are sport-specific. The weight-training program also must be specific in terms of its focus on either muscular strengthening or muscular endurance improvements. Recent evidence suggests that simultaneous training for strength and endurance may have a negative effect on the improvement of strength.[38]

Another aspect of specificity is "practicing perfectly." Considering the amount of force and the stresses involved in weight training, the risk of injury is significantly increased unless the movement and form of the athlete are perfect. An experienced power lifter who had been lifting for more than 15 years and who helped coach many young lifters complained of chronic shoulder pain. When his form was closely scrutinized while he was doing a bench press, it was noted that his painful right shoulder was slightly more externally rotated than the left shoulder, secondary to a 3-degree deviation of the bar from the optimal position. As soon as the position of the bar was corrected, the pain disappeared. This applies to all aspects of training: the sports medicine specialist or professional must be able to analyze critically all aspects of an activity or movement to determine incorrect form and to reduce the risk of injury. Unless athletes practice perfectly, they are predisposing themselves to a greater probability of injury.

FITT Principles for Strength Training

Frequency.   Most strength training is done every other day to allow adequate recovery time between training sessions. Many strength training programs are designed to stress only one area per day and another area on opposite days—for example, upper body on Monday, Wednesday, and Friday and lower body on Tuesday, Thursday, and Saturday. Training for more muscular endurance stresses opposite areas within a single workout, but still alternates between upper- and lower-body exercises. Weight trainers attempt to exercise large muscles first as they adapt to the overload before the smaller weaker muscles fatigue.[5]

Intensity.   Intensity is altered according to the muscle group to be exercised and the purpose of the training. Basically, intensity is designed as it is for interval training. Strength weight training involves few repetitions with maximal or near-maximal weight, whereas endurance weight training involves

Table 3-7. Summary of Advantages of Isokinetic, Isotonic, and Isometric Training Methods

	Type of Training		
Criterion	Isokinetic	Isotonic	Isometric
Rate of Strength Gain	1	1	2
Strength Gain Throughout Range of Motion }	Excellent	Good	Poor
Time per Training Session	2	3	1
Expense	3	2	1
Ease of Performance	2	3	1
Ease of Progress Assessment }	Expensive Equipment Required	Excellent	Dynamometer Required
Adaptability to Specific Movement	1	2	3
Probability of Soreness	Little Soreness	Much Soreness	Little Soreness
Probability of Musculo-skeletal Injury	Slight	Moderate	Slight
Cardiac Risk	Some	Slight	Moderate
Skill Improvement	Some	Some	None

A rating of 1 is superior; 2, intermediate; and 3, inferior.
(Lamb DR: Physiology of Exercise: Responses and Adaptations. p. 280. Macmillan, New York, 1984.)

Table 3-8. Examples of Circuit Training Programs

Duration	10 weeks
Frequency	3 days per week
Circuits/Session	Circuit A = 3, Circuit B = 2
Time/Circuit	Circuit A = 7½ min, Circuit B = 15 min
Total Time/Session	Circuit A = 22½ min, Circuit B = 30 min
Load	40 to 55 % of 1-RM load
Repetitions	As many as possible in 30 seconds
Rest	15 seconds between stations

	Circuit A*		Circuit B
Station	Exercise	Station	Exercise
1	Bench press	1	Running (440 yd)
2	Bent-knee sit-up	2	Push-ups or pull-ups
3	Knee (leg) extension	3	Bent-knee sit-ups
4	Pulldown—lat machine	4	Vertical jumps
5	Back hyperextension	5	Standing (overhead) press
6	Standing (overhead) press	6	Bicycling (3 min)
7	Dead lift	7	Hip stretch
8	Arm curl	8	Rope jumping (1 min)
9	Leg curl (knee flexion)	9	Bent-over rowing
10	Upright rowing	10	Hamstring stretch
		11	Upright rowing
		12	Running (660 yd)

* Modified from Wilmore and co-workers (1978).
(Fox EL: Sports Physiology. © 1979 by Saunders College Publishing/Holt, Rinehart & Winston. Reprinted by permission of CBS College Publishing.)

Table 3-9. Strength Training Exercises for Various Sports

BASEBALL

Incline press
Power clean
Upright row
Triceps extension
Bent-arm pullover
Good morning exercise
Regular squat
Sit-up twisting
Dumbbell swing

BASKETBALL

Bench press
Power clean
Upright row
Dumbbell curl
Lat machine
Lateral arm raise
Bent-arm pullover
Dumbbell swing
Regular squat
Toe raise
Leg curl
Knee extension
Sit-up twisting

FOOTBALL

Bench press
Standing press
Power clean and jerk
Dumbbell curl
Lat machine
Shoulder shrug
Stiff-leg dead lift
Dumbbell swing
Back hyperextension
Regular squat
Knee extension
Sit-up twisting
Neck flexion and
  extension

GOLF

Incline press
Power clean
Upright row
Barbell curl
Dumbbell curl
Parallel bar dip
Stiff-leg dead lift
Dumbbell swing
Regular squat
Hack squat
Sit-up twisting

GYMNASTICS

Incline press
Standing press
Power snatch
Upright row
Dumbbell curl
Lat machine
Parallel bar dip
Triceps extension
Lateral arm raise
Dumbbell swing
Back hyperextension
Hack squat

HOCKEY

Incline press
Power clean
Upright row
Dumbbell curl
Lat machine
Parallel bar dip
Triceps extension
Shoulder shrug
Good morning exercise
Dumbbell swing
Hack squat
Knee extension
Sit-up twisting
Neck flexion and
  extension

MOUNTAIN CLIMBING

Incline press
Upright row
Barbell curl
Lat machine
Triceps extension
Shoulder shrug
Stiff-leg dead lift
Hack squat
Toe raise
Leg curl
Knee extension
Sit-up

ROWING

Bench press
Power clean
Upright row
Lat machine
Dumbbell curl
Parallel bar dip
Bent-arm pullover
Good morning exercise

Back hyperextension
Regular squat
Hack squat
Sit-up

SKIING

Incline press
Upright row
Dumbbell curl
Lat machine
Triceps extension
Parallel bar dip
Shoulder shrug
Good morning exercise
Dumbbell swing
Hack squat
Knee extension
Leg curl
Toe raise
Sit-up twisting

SOCCER

Incline press
Power clean
Bent-over row
Barbell curl
Parallel bar dip
Bent-arm pullover
Stiff-leg dead lift
Dumbbell swing
Regular squat
Knee extension
Sit-up twisting
Neck flexion and
  extension

SWIMMING

Back Stroke

Press behind neck
Incline press
Upright row
Lat machine
Lateral arm raise
Shoulder shrug
Dumbbell swing
Hack squat
Knee extension
Horizontal leg raise

Breast Stroke

Bench press
Power clean
Upright row

(O'Shea JP: Scientific Principles and Methods of Strength Fitness. pp. 92–93. Addison Wesley, Reading, 1976.)

(continued)

Table 3-9. *(Continued)*

Lat machine
Triceps extension
Bent-arm pullover
Dumbbell swing
Back hyperextension
Hack squat
Leg curl
Horizontal leg raise

Butterfly

Bench press
Press behind neck
Power clean
Lat machine
Triceps extension,
  using lat machine
Bent-arm pullover
Dumbbell swing
Hack squat
Leg curl
Horizontal leg raise

Free Style

Bench press
Standing press
Upright row
Bent-over row
Triceps extension
Parallel bar dip
Bent-arm pullover
Stiff-leg dead lift
Back hyperextension
Hack squat
Horizontal leg lift

TENNIS

Incline press
Standing press
Upright row
Dumbbell curl
Reverse curl
Triceps extension
Lateral arm raise
Shoulder shrug
Stiff-leg dead lift
Dumbbell swing
Hack squat
Sit-up twisting

TRACK AND FIELD

Discus and Shot Put

Bench press
Incline press

Standing press
Power clean
Barbell curl
Tricep extension
Good morning exercise
Dumbbell swing
Regular squat
Knee extension
Sit-up twisting

Distance Running

Bench press
Power clean
Upright row
Dumbbell curl
Stiff-leg dead lift
Hack squat
Straight-arm pullover
Toe raise
Sit-up twisting

High Jump

Incline press
Bench press
Power clean
Dumbbell curl
Bent-arm pullover
Hack squat
Knee extension
Toe raise
Sit-up

Hurdling

Incline press
Power clean
Bent-over row
Lat machine
Dumbbell swing
Hack squat
Toe raise
Knee extension
Leg curl
Sit-up twisting

Javelin

Incline press
Standing press
Power clean
Triceps extension
Bent-arm pullover
Shoulder shrug
Hack squat
Toe raise

Leg curl
Knee extension
Sit-up twisting

Long Jump

Incline press
Power clean
Dumbbell curl
Triceps extension
Bent-arm pullover
Hack squat
Knee extension
Horizontal leg raise

Pole Vault

Bench press
Incline press
Power clean
Upright row
Lateral arm raise
Bent-arm pullover
Shoulder shrug
Back hyperextension
Hack squat
Sit-up twisting

Sprinting

Bench press
Power clean
Dumbbell curl
Good morning exercise
Back hyperextension
Hack squat
Leg curl
Knee extension
Toe raise

WRESTLING

Bench press
Standing press
Power clean
Bent-over row
Dumbbell curl
Lat machine
Triceps extension
Parallel bar dip
Good morning exercise
Back hyperextension
Regular squat
Knee extension
Sit-up twisting
Neck flexion and
  extension

more repetitions at a lower weight. Specificity of training as it relates to the athlete's event should dictate the intensity of exercise.

Time or Duration. Because a muscle needs to have adequate recovery to perform optimally, most weight training workouts last several hours, while the actual time of movement may be only several minutes. From this standpoint, weight training per se does nothing to improve the athlete's aerobic capacity.

Type of Training. There are several considerations for the type of weight training prescribed to make it sports-specific. The use of eccentric or concentric muscle contraction is an important consideration. Many activities involve both concentric and eccentric contractions. Through careful analysis of the activity, specific weight-training exercises can be incorporated into the training program to simulate the strength needs of the activity. Whether to use isometrics, isotonics, or isokinetics as the choice of training mode requires careful consideration.

Isometrics. Isometrics involve a static contraction with little or no joint movement. The contraction should be at least 75 percent of the maximal voluntary contraction or greater and should be held 2 to 8 seconds.[8,37] Longer periods of maximal static contraction will promote a Valsalva's maneuver, leading to increased blood pressure, and should be avoided. Recovery should be between 2 and 3 minutes between contractions; normally there are six to eight repetitions. It is important to perform isometric contractions at more than one joint angle, because strengthening occurs only where the muscle is stressed.[8,37]

Isotonics. Isotonics involve a concentric and eccentric movement of a preset resistance through a range of motion. The resistance can be constant (free-weight training), variable (Nautilus), eccentric (lowering a weight while the muscle lengthens and allowing a person or machine to perform the concentric movement), or manual (proprioceptive neuromuscular facilitation, PNF).[2] Isotonic exercise normally involves 1 to 10 repetitions of an exercise: 3 to 4 sets of each exercise with 5 to 10 minutes of recovery between sets. Isotonic workouts are normally done three days per week.[5] A relatively new form of isotonic training, plyometric training, involves implosion training: a muscle is suddenly loaded and forced to stretch before contraction can occur (e.g., jumping from a bench down to the surface and back up to the bench).[2] These activities are used a great deal by track and field athletes to increase their jumping ability, but they are not without substantial risk of knee and back injury. More scientific research is required to assess the merit of plyometric training.[2]

Isokinetics. Isokinetic exercise is exercise through range of motion with the speed of movement controlled; thus the resistance accommodates through the force applied. Because the speed can be controlled, specific sport-related velocities can be adapted and training can be specifically at these speeds. Isokinetic exercises have a significantly lower risk of injury because the athlete, not a machine, controls the resistance. The major drawback to isokinetic training is the expense of the equipment, which prohibits many athletes from using it. Sports medicine professionals can use isokinetics in both rehabilitation and training of athletes.

Table 3-7 presents a comparison of advantages and disadvantages of all three of these strengthening programs.

CIRCUIT TRAINING

In circuit training, the athlete completes a number of repetitions at a given station before moving to the next station. The number of stations regulates the number of exercises. The length of time at each station and the time to get to the next station can be regulated, and the exercises that comprise the circuit can vary to fit the needs of the athlete. One circuit equals one round of all stations. The number of circuits can be varied to suit the requirements of the sport.

Circuit training allows a number of people to exercise simultaneously and allows the development of muscular endurance. Table 3-8 shows two examples of circuit training programs, one for strength development and one for endurance training. Note that the stations tend to alternate between arms, back, and legs to allow for some recovery.

Table 3-9 presents suggestions for weight-training exercises for 25 different sports and athletic activities. Other exercises may be used, but these suggestions stress the major areas where sport-specific strengthening exercises may help to improve performance.

SUMMARY

The general training principles of overload, specificity, individualized prescription, and FITT apply to all forms of training. Sports medicine professionals should be familiar with the athlete's activities to assist the coach and athlete in obtaining maximum benefit from training. As sports medicine continues to grow and as our knowledge of training is increased through research and experience, athletes will benefit even more from training methods.

REFERENCES

1. Åstrand PO, Rodahl K: Textbook of Work Physiology. McGraw–Hill, New York, 1977
2. Brooks GA, Fahey TD: Exercise Physiology: Human Bioenergentics and Its Applications, Wiley, New York, 1984
3. Fox EL: Sports Physiology. WB Saunders, Philadelphia, 1984

4. Fox EL, Mathews DK: The Physiological Basis of Physical Education and Athletics. WB Saunders, Philadelphia, 1983
5. Lamb DR: Physiology of Exercise: Responses and Adaptations. Macmillan, New York, 1984
6. Maglischo EW: Swimming Faster. Mayfield, Palo Alto, 1982
7. McArdle WD, Katch FI, Katch VL: Exercise Physiology: Energy, Nutrition, and Human Performance. Lea and Febiger, Philadelphia, 1981
8. O'Shea JP: Scientific Principles and Methods of Strength Fitness. Addison Wesley, Reading, 1976
9. Wilmore JH: Athletic Training and Physical Fitness. Allyn and Bacon, Boston, 1984
10. American College of Sports Medicine: Guidelines for Graded Exercise Testing and Exercise Prescription. Lea and Febiger, Philadelphia, 1980
11. Fox EL, Mathews DK: Interval Training: Conditioning for Sport and General Fitness. WB Saunders, Philadelphia, 1974
12. Cardus D: Exercise testing: methods and uses. Exerc Sports Sci Rev 6:59, 1978
13. Ellestad MH, Cooke BM, Greenberg PS: Stress testing: clinical applications and predictive capacity. Prog Cardiovas Dis 21:431, 1979
14. Nagle FJ: Physiological assessment of maximal performance. Exerc Sports Sci Rev 1:313, 1973
15. Jones NL, Campbell EJ: Clinical Exercise Testing. WB Saunders, Philadelphia, 1982
16. Ellestad MH: Stress Testing: Principles and Practice. FA Davis, Philadelphia, 1984
17. Mellerowicz H, Smodlaka VN: Ergometry: Basics of Medical Exercise Testing. Urban and Schwarzenberg, Baltimore, 1981
18. Åstrand PO: Work Tests with the Bicycle Ergometer. Monark–Cresent AB Varberg, Sweden
19. Bowerman, WJ, Harris WE: Jogging. Grosset and Dunlap, New York, 1977
20. Cooper KH: Aerobics. M Evans, New York, 1968
21. Cooper KH: The Aerobics Way. M Evans, New York, 1977
22. Pollack ML, Cureton TK, Greninger L: Effects of frequency of training on working capacity, cardiovascular function and body composition of adult men. Med Sci Sports Exerc 1:70, 1969
23. Pollack ML: The quantification of endurance training programs. Exerc Sports Sci Rev 1:155, 1973
24. Brynteson P, Sinning WE: The effects of training frequencies on the retention of cardiovascular fitness. Med Sci Sports Exerc 5:29, 1973
25. Pollack ML, Gettman, LR, Milesis CA et al: Effects of frequency and duration of training on attrition and incidence of injury. Med Sci Sports Exerc 9:31, 1977
26. Hickson RC, Rosenkoether MA: Reduced training frequencies and the maintenance of increased aerobic power. Med Sci Sports Exerc 13:13, 1981
27. Hickson RC, Kanakis C, Davies JR et al: Reduced training duration effects on aerobic power, endurance and cardiac growth. J Appl Physiol 53:225, 1982
28. Wilson PK, Bell CW, Norton AC: Rehabilitation of the Heart and Lungs. Beckman Instruments, Fullerton, CA, 1980
29. Wasserman K, Whipp BJ: Exercise physiology in health and disease. Am Rev Respir Dis 112:219, 1975
30. Stamford BA, Weltman A, Moffat R et al: Exercise recovery above and below the anaerobic threshold following maximal work. J Appl Physiol 51:840, 1981
31. Fox EL, Bartels RL, Billings CE et al: Frequency and duration of interval training programs and changes in aerobic power. J Appl Physiol 38:481, 1975

32. Fox EL: Physical training: methods and effects. Orthop Clin North Am 8:533, 1977
33. Furman G: Effects of clinical bed rest for seven days on physical performance. Acta Med Scand 205:389, 1979
34. Houston ME, Bentzen H, Larsen H: Interrelationship between skeletal muscle adaptation and performance as studied by detraining and retraining. Acta Physiol Scand 105:163, 1979
35. Saltin B, Blomquist G, Mitchell JH et al: Response of exercise after bedrest and training. Circulation 38, suppl. 7:1, 1968
36. Pedersen PK, Jørgensen K: Maximal oxygen uptake in young women with training inactivity and retraining. Med Sci Sports Exerc 10:233, 1978
37. Clarke DH: Adaptations in strength and musular endurance resulting from exercise. Exerc Sports Sci Rev 1:73, 1973
38. Hickson RC: Interference of strength development by simultaneously training for strength and endurance. Eur J Appl Physiol 45:255, 1980

4 | Physiological Basis of Warm-up and Cool-down

John S. Leard
Janet E. Guilfoyle

For some time, it has been generally accepted that a brief warm-up period prior to a maximal exercise effort enhances an individual's performance and decreases his or her risk of injury. More recently, the concept of a cool-down period following an activity has been encouraged to enhance the individual's ability to recover from a strenuous workout.

There is confusion as to the reasons for warm-up and cool-down and what exercises should be included in each type of session. In this chapter we discuss the physiological basis of warm-up and cool-down activities and give examples of specific exercises that could be included in a routine.

WARM-UP

Warm-up exercises are designed to increase the temperature of the muscles, usually by movement, to prepare them for strenuous work. The two basic types of warm-up exercises are general and specific.[1]

General Warm-up

General warm-up prepares the major muscle groups for activity through active movement. The exercises increase the body temperature through muscular contraction. Jumping rope and calisthenics are examples of general warm-up exercises. Any exercise not directly associated with the nervous or muscular components of the expected activity is considered a general warm-up exercise.

Specific Warm-up

Specific warm-up concentrates on the muscle groups involved in the expected activity. Specific warm-up not only increases the temperature of the specific muscle groups, it elicits the increased neuromuscular transmission of impulses to those muscles.[1] This response allows for better recruitment of the motor units utilized in a specific skill. A specific warm-up exercise closely simulates the skill an individual is to perform. For example, a specific warm-up technique for a shotputter would be to go through a series of partial and/or submaximal throwing motions prior to competition.

Effects of Warm-up

The increase in body temperature produced by warm-up exercises results in a variety of physiological effects. The ability of hemoglobin to release oxygen into the muscle tissues is enhanced,[1,2] allowing for a more rapid metabolic process within the muscles and an increase in the functional efficiency of the working muscle units. A vasodilation response is elicited in the muscle units, resulting in increased blood flow to the vascular beds of the working muscles. The increased blood flow in turn decreases blood viscosity, thus enhancing the functional efficiency of the working muscle groups. As blood flow increases, more of the blood elements needed for metabolism circulate. The increased blood flow also may decrease the buildup of products resulting from exercise.[3]

Muscular contraction at elevated temperatures occurs more quickly and forcefully, allowing the individual to perform complex movements in a coordinated manner.[2] This ability is enhanced further by increased transmissions of neuromuscular impulses to the working muscle groups.[4] The increased ability of neuromuscular impulses to travel to major muscle groups involved could increase the individual's ability to react to sudden movement or direction changes.

The cardiorespiratory system is allowed time to adapt to the demands of maximal physical effort. This has a positive influence on physical parameters such as blood pressure and the ability of the heart to circulate blood to the body parts needing it most.[5]

Data supporting the belief that warm-up decreases the chance for injury are not substantial at this time, but increased blood flow to muscles has a positive influence on elasticity.[6] Increased elasticity enhances mechanical functioning and the ability of working muscle units to adapt to changes in length. It seems safe to assume that increased elasticity and improved reaction time enhance the individual's ability to react to the stresses of a particular activity and have a positive influence on decreasing injury occurrence.

The psychological effects of adequate warm-up cannot be discounted. Warm-up allows the athlete to become mentally prepared for the activity and may increase the quality of the performance. Many athletes use their warm-up time to go through the activity mentally: they find that mental imagery helps them to react more quickly when performing the activity. Others use the time to concentrate and eliminate any distractions that may influence their performance.

Goals of Warm-up

A good warm-up routine can be done in many ways, as long as four basic goals are accomplished:

1. The blood flow to the muscles being exercised should increase, raising muscle temperature and resulting in the previously outlined physiological effects.
2. Respiration should increase, allowing the respiratory system to meet the increased demand for oxygen.
3. Pulse rate should increase, enabling oxygen-filled blood to be carried to the muscles.
4. Active movements of the joints of the body should allow an increase in synovial fluid production and decrease stress on the articular surfaces.

Duration and Intensity

The duration and intensity of the warm-up session are important considerations. It is unreasonable to assign a specific amount of time that applies to any warm-up session. Duration is based on the individual's level of fitness, the environmental temperature and humidity, and the type of activity.

A good indicator that warm-up is sufficient is the stimulation of the sweating mechanism: sweating indicates that the body temperature has increased and therefore the desired physiological responses have occurred. A well-conditioned athlete needs a more intense and possibly longer warm-up to attain an adequate increase in temperature. If the warm-up is performed in a cool environment, more activity is necessary to build up heat in the extremities because peripheral circulation is decreased to maintain the core temperature. In a warm environment, peripheral vasodilation occurs in the extremities to disperse the heat and sufficient warm-up is achieved more quickly.

Once warm-up is achieved, it must be maintained. During practice, stretches in inactivity could allow cooling. If the muscles must be warm to perform optimally, the athlete and coach should adjust the warm-up to maintain body temperature. Warm-up should not be done too far in advance of the anticipated activity, because body temperature returns to normal after approximately 45 minutes of rest.

Warm-up should not be so intense that the athlete fatigues more rapidly during the activity. This is influenced by the individual's level of fitness. The warm-up should achieve the desired physiological changes without minimizing performance.[7] For each specific athletic event, the amount of warm-up must be adjusted to balance intensity and duration to improve performance.

Warm-up Routine

A general warm-up routine usually incorporates jogging, calisthenics, and stretching. Contracting and relaxing muscles rhythmically is the next most effective type of exercise to increase heat in the muscles. Stretching exercises *do not* warm up the muscles. Stretching involves the lengthening and relaxation of the musculotendinous units and stretching of other soft tissues supporting the joints. If stretching is incorporated into a warm-up, it should follow the increase in temperature of the body part that will be stretched. Warm-up increases the elasticity of the soft tissue around the joint and makes the exercises easier and more profitable.[6] Static or proprioceptive neuromuscular facilitation (PNF) stretching techniques should be used to stretch the musculature. Ballistic types of stretching increase the risk of tearing the muscle and firing the stretch reflex.[8] Flexibility exercises should not cause pain, only a gentle stretching sensation. The individual should be aware of his or her range of joint motion and not try to perform stretching exercises that would overstretch and cause tearing of soft tissue. Flexibility exercises are most suited for the cool-down routine, when the muscles are already warm and therefore more flexible.

The general warm-up routine should work all the major joints of the body. Exercises should begin slowly and gradually increase in intensity and range of joint movement. The general warm-up could emphasize certain muscle groups according to the activity that follows. For instance, in a general warm-up for tennis, extra exercises for the shoulder complex and upper extremities of the dominant hand could be incorporated into the routine. A warm-up should not be primarily used to strengthen certain muscle groups, but this could be a secondary goal of the routine.

The following is an example of a general warm-up routine for running.

1. **Walking:** Begin at a normal pace and gradually increase speed and stride length. Dress warmly enough for the environment in which you are working. Concentrate on deep, regular breathing and a heel-to-toe walking pattern.
2. **Walk-jog:** Alternate jogging for approximately 220 yards with walking for *approximately 20* yards. Do this two to three times. While walking, begin to shake your legs and arms with gradually increasing force. This type of vigorous movement increases circulation without causing stress to the joints.
3. **Active Motion:** Begin movements of muscles joint by joint.
   A. **Neck**—Gently move in flexion, extension, lateral flexion, and rotation. Perform neck circles in both directions. Do this slowly. Gradually increase the range with each repetition. Start this in the walk cycle of the walk–jog exercise.
   B. **Shoulder**—Shrug your shoulders, then bring them back, ad-

ducting the scapula. Depress the scapula and follow by protraction. Continue the shoulder circles, beginning with small movements and gradually increasing range and rhythm. Perform in both directions. Do this while walking or standing.

C. **Shoulder**—Adduct the shoulders to 90 percent and make a fist with each hand. Begin rotating your arms forward in small circles with your elbow extended. Gradually increase the size of the circles until there are wide sweeping circles that cross in front of the body. Repeat the exercise in each direction. The hand can be alternately opened and closed while performing the shoulder circles. Do this while walking or standing.

D. **Trunk**—Standing with your arms abducted to 90° and your feet shoulder-width apart, alternately rotate to the left and to the right. Begin with a small range and a slow rhythm. Gradually increase the range, being careful care not to move too quickly, which could tear soft tissue.

E. **Legs**—Lying on your back with both knees flexed, extend one leg and hold it 6 inches above the ground with the foot plantar flexed. Flex the hip and knee of the same leg while dorsiflexing the ankle. Repeat with the other leg.

4. **Calisthenics:** Perform jumping jacks to maintain the breathing and pulse rates attained during the walk–job cycle. This is also a general warm-up for the arm and leg musculature.

Additional warm-up exercises can be interspersed or substituted for the ones in the routine. The exercise period could be followed by flexibility exercises, because the muscles will be warm enough to be stretched. Jogging would follow, beginning slowly and gradually increasing to performance level. Intensity and duration are determined by fitness level and desired physiological responses.

A specific warm-up routine incorporates the partial and submaximal motions of the event. A baseball pitcher's warm-up usually consists of throwing the ball, beginning with a short distance and gradually increasing distance and intensity to the activity level. A variation would be to begin with short-distance throwing with only the elbow and wrist and gradually to increase the distance of each throw and incorporate the shoulder and trunk rotation movements.

An example of a specific warm-up for tennis is to start with easy hitting close to the net or practice wall and gradually increase the distance from the net as well as the force with which the ball is hit. Next, the service is practiced by going through the motions several times without striking the ball. When the ball is used, the force begins at one-fourth the normal amount and gradually is increased to full force. Even following a proper general warm-up, the athlete should never begin all-out playing. The specific warm-up allows the muscles used during the activity time to adjust to the stress they must withstand.

Specific warm-up routines usually follow the general warm-up, so flexibility exercises may have been performed already. Pitching, like most sports that require an overhead motion of the arm, requires "excessive" external rotation (120 degrees or more) to decrease stress on the shoulder and elbow. It is theorized that the lack of this excessive motion causes many of the overuse types of injuries seen at the shoulder.[9] Because of this, flexibility exercises of the shoulder girdle should be stressed with these types of sports. Again, flexibility exercises can take place in the warm-up or cool-down period, but the muscles must be warm before stretching begins.

COOL-DOWN

The period immediately following exercise is termed the "cool-down session." "It is believed that since intense muscular exercise results in the production of lactate, which inhibits the rate of glycolysis and free fatty acid mobilization, then the removal of lactate after high-intensity exercise may be critical for subsequent performance. Several studies do indicate that lactate removal is enhanced during recovery by moderate aerobic exercise."[3] This exercise also helps to aid venous blood return to the heart by the pumping action of the muscles, thus preventing pooling of blood in the extremities.[10] Other studies show that rest following exercise results in a faster net heart rate of return to a baseline level of net oxygen uptake.[10]

Katch and co-workers[10] discussed the advantage of "active" versus "passive" recovery from supramaximal exercise. Active recovery incorporates some type of submaximal aerobic activity following strenuous exercise. Passive recovery does not incorporate any type of submaximal activity; it is primarily a period of rest following exercise. They suggested that active recovery is most advantageous because blood lactate levels decrease more readily in active versus passive recovery.

During aerobic activity, blood flow to internal organs is decreased to allow for maximal circulation to the working muscles. It has been suggested that during aerobic recovery, rather than the traditional metabolic process of gluconeogenesis in the liver, the blood lactate is oxidized by the working muscles for ATP production and that the ability of the working muscles to oxidize the lactate is enhanced by the recruitment of slow-twitch, high-oxidative muscle fibers.[3]

During active recovery, the ability to metabolize lactate through the working muscles is influenced by the rate of blood flow and concentration of lactate in the blood. If high-oxidative, slow-twitch fibers are recruited during an aerobic recovery session, lactate will be taken up for metabolism more efficiently. This leads to a decreased blood level following exercise. An individual's aerobic fitness level has a positive influence on aerobic recovery levels and thus also influences lactate uptake.

Active cool-down and decreasing blood lactate levels may have a direct influence on the individual's ability to return to maximal exercise, as does aerobic fitness levels. An adequate cool-down session that incorporates submaximal aerobic work could have a positive influence on an individual's ability to resume physical activity after a maximal effort.[10]

Goals of Cool-down

The goals of a cool-down routine are

1. to reduce the blood lactate levels as quickly as possible to increase recovery.
2. to allow the heart rate, respiration, and other bodily functions to adjust to the change in activity level.
3. to increase or maintain muscular flexibility by stretching warm muscles.

Cool-down Routine

A cool-down session could incorporate walking, jogging, or other low-level aerobic activities and flexibility exercise into the recovery period. The two types of activities could be alternated to produce physiological benefits of both active and passive recovery and the benefits of stretching a warmed muscle.

Duration

Cool-down sessions can last as long as the heart rate is elevated above the resting heart rate level. Usually, cool-down ends when the athlete feels recovered and the heart rate is at a reasonable level relative to the resting pulse.

Benefits of Cool-down

Some individuals have reported that muscle soreness, which sometimes follows maximal effort, is eliminated by incorporating a cool-down period into a workout. The literature does not directly support this claim. There are several theories for delayed muscle soreness, including lactic acid accumulation, the spasm theory, the torn tissue theory, and the connective tissue theory. Recent studies indicate that muscular or connective tissue microtears are the cause.[11] If this is true a cool-down session would not appear to have any direct effect on muscular soreness.

Others claim that they are less fatigued the day after a workout with a cool-down. This may be explained by the lactate removal and subsequent increase in the rate of glycolysis and mobilization of free fatty acids.[3] In turn, this process could have a positive influence in subsequent exercise performances.

SUMMARY

Warm-up, which prepares the individual for exercise by raising the temperature of the body, can decrease injuries and increase performance. Stretching exercises do not have to be a major part of a warm-up session: they are probably more suited to cool-down, when the muscle is warm. Cool-down enables the body slowly to return to its resting state and prepares the muscles to work optimally in subsequent exercise.

REFERENCES

1. Shellock FG: Physiological benefits of warm-up. Phys Sports Med 11:134, 1983
2. Davies C, Young K: Effect of temperature on the contractile properties and muscle power of triceps surae in humans. J Appl Physiol 55:191, 1983
3. Weltman A, Stamford B, Moffatt R, Katch VL: Exercise recovery, lactate removal, and subsequent high intensity exercise performance. Research Quarterly 48:786, 1977
4. Roca J: Effects of warming up on reaction time and movement in the lower extremities. Int J Sports Psychol, 11:165, 1980
5. Barnard RJ, Gardner GW, Diaco NV et al: Cardiovascular response to sudden strenuous exercise-heart rate, blood pressure, and ECG. J Appl Physiol 34:833, 1973
6. Lehmann JF, Massock AJ, Warren CG et al: Effect of therapeutic temperatures on tendon extensibility. Arch Phys Med Rehabil 51:481, 1970
7. Genovely H, Stanford BA: Effects of prolonged warm-up exercise above and below anaerobic threshold on maximal performance. Eur J Appl Physiol Occup Physiol 48:323, 1982
8. Bennet R: Principles of therapeutic exercise. In Licht A (ed): Therapeutic Exercise. Waverly Press, Baltimore, 1965
9. Norwood LA, DelPizzo W, Jobe FW et al: Anterior shoulder pain in baseball pitchers. Am J Sports Med 16:103, 1978
10. Katch V, Gilliam T, Weltman A: Active vs passive recovery from short term supramaximal exercise. Research Quarterly 49:153, 1978
11. Francis KT: Delayed muscle soreness—a review. J Orthop Sports Phys Ther 5:10, 1983

5 | Nutritional Requirements for Athletes

Mary Bauman

Athletes commonly develop an interest in nutrition because they wish to maximize energy for training and competition. Because they are so interested in nutrition, they are uniquely vulnerable to nutritional misinformation alleging to improve performance.[1]

Just about every nutrient has at one time or another been purported to improve performance. The fact is, no single nutrient in excess of what is supplied by a well-balanced diet, no special foods, protein powders, or amino acid supplements are needed. Such substances do not enhance physical performance and in many cases may actually impair the athlete's potential by interfering with the optimal functioning of the body.

Poor nutrition, on the other hand, can adversely affect an athlete's performance. A nutritionally adequate diet is therefore crucial for competitors wishing to achieve their full athletic potential. A nutritionally adequate diet is one that provides the recommended daily allowances (RDA) for all essential nutrients and energy to meet the body's needs during daily activities, training, and competition.

The nutritional needs of athletes are essentially the same as those of non-athletes in that the 50 or so nutrients required for top performance are the same as those required for everyday activities. The difference is in the quantity of nutrients needed. Endurance athletes, for example, may have increased needs for calories, fluids, and certain vitamins and minerals. All of these needs, however, can be met through the consumption of a well-balanced diet. Even the needs of athletes involved in the most intensive training and competitive sched-

Table 5-1. Recommended Daily Intake of Four Major Food Groups

Food Group	Serving Size	Recommended Servings	Major Nutrient Contributions
Milk			
Milk	1 cup	Teens: 4 or more	Calcium
Yogurt	1 cup	Adults: 2 or more	Riboflavin
Cheese*	1½ oz		Protein
Cottage Cheese*	2 cups		
Ice Cream	1¾ cups		
Pudding	1 cup		
Meat and Meat Substitutes			
Meat (lean)	2 oz	2 or more	Protein
Fish	2 oz		Iron
Poultry	2 oz		Niacin
Eggs	2		Thiamin
Cheese*	2 oz		
Cottage cheese*	½ cup		
Nuts, seeds	⅓–1 cup		
Peanut butter	4 tbs		
Dry beans, peas	1 cup		
Fruit and vegetables			
Fresh, frozen, canned, dried, or juices	½ cup or standard portion, such as 1 medium piece of fruit	4 or more	Vitamin A Vitamin C
Bread and cereals			
Bread	1 slice	4 or more	Carbohydrate
Cereals	½–1 cup		Thiamin
Rolls, muffins	1 med		Iron
Pasta	½ cup		Niacin
Rice	½ cup		

* Cheese should count as a serving of milk *or* meat, not both.

ule can be met if reasonable food choices are made. Foods with a high nutrient density (high nutrient-to-calorie ratio) should be seleted over less nutrient-dense foods. Foods such as dairy products, meats, fruits, vegetables, breads, and cereals have high nutrient-to-calorie ratios; most snack foods, such as cakes, pies, cookies, soft drinks, and other processed foods, have low ratios and are less nutrient-dense.

The minimum number of servings of nutrient-dense foods that are the basis of a nutritionally adequate diet are shown in Table 5-1. Since the minimum number of recommended servings provide only about 1,200 calories, additional servings from each food group can be added as necessary to satisfy an individual's caloric requirements. Indeed, athletes in training may need to consume as many as eight or more servings from each of the fruit–vegetable and bread–cereal groups. All athletes who consume the minimum number of recommended servings from these four major food groups can be confident that their requirements for all essential nutrients except calories are being met. Two other exceptions may be in the need for iron and calcium.

Making appropriate food choices is a difficult task, yet if they are to perform at their best, athletes must learn to devote the same effort to maintaining good nutrition as they do to regular training and competition.

NUTRIENT NEEDS FOR ATHLETES

Athletes require six major nutrients for optimal sports performance: carbohydrates, proteins, fats, vitamins, minerals, and water. Three of these nutrients—carbohydrates, proteins, and fats—are capable of supplying energy to the body's cells. During exercise, a combination of these nutrients is used to fuel the working muscles. The proportion that each contributes to the total energy needs of the muscles depends largely on the type, duration, and intensity of the exercise performed.

Carbohydrates

The major function of carbohydrates in the body is to supply energy for all metabolic reactions and the growth and maintenance of body cells. Carbohydrates are the principal source of energy for the red blood cells, cells of the central nervous system, and muscle cells during short-term exercise. In more prolonged exercise, carbohydrates are used in combination with fats.

There are two main types of dietary carbohydrates: simple and complex. Simple carbohydrates are made up of one or two sugar molecules, while complex carbohydrates are composed of many sugar molecules linked together in long chains. Examples of simple carbohydrates are the sweets in our diet (e.g., cakes, pies, cookies, candy, jellies, honey, soft drinks). Fruit and milk also contain simple carbohydrates but are more nutritious in that they have a higher nutrient density than other simple sugars. Complex carbohydrates include whole grains, cereals, potatoes, breads, pasta, vegetables, and some fruits. These nutrient-dense foods supply many more vitamins, minerals, protein, and fiber than do most simple carbohydrates.

Glucose, a simple carbohydrate, is the major product formed by the breakdown of most dietary carbohydrates in the process of digestion and is the most readily available source of energy for all body cells. Each gram of carbohydrate can be broken down to supply four calories of energy. One-half cup of spaghetti (22 g carbohydrates), for example, can provide 88 calories of energy. If not used immediately for energy, dietary carbohydrates can be stored in the liver and muscles as glycogen (a long chain of glucose molecules). There is, however, a limited storage capacity for glycogen (approximately 80 to 90 g in the liver, 350 g in muscles[2]) and amounts in excess of immediate energy needs or storage capacity will quickly be converted to and stored as fat.

Glucose and glycogen are particularly important to athletes since they are the form of carbohydrates used to supply energy to the working muscles. During the first few minutes of exercise, blood glucose is the major fuel source. As exercise progresses, the increasing energy demands of the muscles are met by the muscle's own glycogen supply. The quantity of glycogen used depends largely on the intensity and duration of the exercise performed; the greater the intensity and the longer the duration of the high-intensity exercise, the more glycogen is used. Because glycogen stores are limited, they cannot sustain prolonged strenuous exercise indefinitely. During a marathon, cross-country skiing, or long-distance cycling, for example, the energy demands of the active muscles are extreme and could result in depletion of the glycogen supply within 2 or 3 hours. Sports that involve repeated bouts of high-intensity effort, such as basketball, football, or soccer, can also impose a significant drain on the muscle glycogen stores.[3] When glycogen stores are depleted, the athlete's performance is drastically impaired. In a marathon, this phenomenon is known as "hitting the wall." When the muscles run out of energy for contraction, the runner is forced to slow down. As discussed later, ingestion of additional carbohydrate during long-term competitive events can improve endurance performance by preventing early depletion of the body's glycogen stores.

In contrast, during short-term, high-intensity events, such as a 1,500-m run or a giant slalom ski race, the quantity of glycogen used is much less. Athletes involved in these events generally have sufficient glycogen stores to maintain optimal performance provided they eat a normal balanced diet adequate in carbohydrates.

Most athletes in training should consume a diet that provides 50 to 55 percent of their calories from carbohydrates. Endurance athletes, however, may experience a gradual depletion of carbohydrate stores with successive days of strenuous training and therefore should eat a diet higher in carbohydrates. For these athletes, a diet that provides as much as 70 percent of the days' calories from carbohydrates will help to replenish glycogen stores and ensure that energy needs are met.

Complex carbohydrates provide fiber, water, and other valuable nutrients, whereas simple carbohydrates are often high in fat and contain few, if any, other nutrients. In addition, complex carbohydrates promote glycogen storage better than simple sugars.[4] For these reasons it is recommended that athletes choose a diet higher in complex rather than simple carbohydrates.

Fats

Fats are a concentrated source of energy that can be used by all body cells except the red blood cells and the cells of the nervous system, which must rely strictly on glucose. Each gram of fat supplies 9 calories—more than twice the amount of energy from carbohydrate or protein. The main source of this energy is fatty acids. Fatty acids, like carbohydrates, are a major fuel source for the muscles during prolonged exercise. Fats are also necessary to absorb fat-soluble vitamins (A, D, E, and K), to protect body organs, and to maintain the structure of cell membranes. In addition, fat, rather than carbohydrate, is the preferred fuel source for the heart.

Fats are important energy sources because of their tremendous storage capacity compared with carbohydrates. A highly trained male athlete, for example, who weighs 65 kg and has 6 percent body fat would have approximately 4 kg of fat, which is the equivalent of 36,000 calories. In contrast, carbohydrate stores can contribute only about 1,400 to 2,000 calories to the energy needs of an athlete. Conditions that favor the use of fat for energy help to protect the limited carbohydrate stores, which are the required energy source for certain tissues. Thus, through their sparing effect on the carbohydrate stores, fats have the ability to enhance the time for which prolonged strenuous exercise can be sustained.

Although the supply of fat is almost unlimited, the ability of the muscles to utilize it for energy is not.[5] An important factor governing fatty acid utilization during prolonged exercise is the individual's state of training. Athletes well trained for endurance events use more fat and less carbohydrate than less-trained individuals. Indeed, endurance athletes can derive as much as 75 percent of their total energy requirement from fatty acids during prolonged strenuous activity.[6]

Because it takes at least 30 minutes from the start of exercise for fatty acids to be utilized in large amounts, they are of less significant benefit to strength and power athletes or to any athlete involved in high-intensity events lasting less than 30 minutes. The energy derived during these events comes primarily from carbohydrates.

Although a minimal amount of fat in the diet is important, most individuals, athletes included, consume more than is necessary. A high-fat diet can potentially hinder optimal sports performance. Because fatty foods are generally low in nutrient density, a high-fat diet could deprive the athlete of essential nutrients. In addition, when dietary intake of fat is high, carbohydrate intake is usually insufficient to maintain adequate levels of glycogen in the muscles. It is therefore recommended that fat intake be restricted to less than 30 to 35 percent of daily calories. To achieve the recommended intake, athletes should avoid or limit rich desserts; select low-fat dairy products; limit butter, cream, and other high-fat foods; and choose lean meats, poultry, and fish over beef, pork, cold cuts, bacon, and sausage. Individuals with high caloric requirements should obtain their extra calories by consuming additional servings of breads, cereals, fruits, and vegetables, which contain negligible amounts of fat.

Proteins

Proteins are essential nutrients that have many important and diverse functions. Proteins are needed throughout the body to build and repair all cells and tissues, including the internal organs, muscles, blood cells, bones, and skin. Proteins are also components of enzymes and some hormones that help to regulate many essential body reactions.

Proteins, like carbohydrates, can supply 4 calories of energy per gram and are used for this purpose when the body is unable to obtain enough calories from carbohydrates and fats. If used for energy, however, protein will no longer be available to perform other necessary functions.

While proteins do not normally contribute to the energy needs of healthy individuals at rest, they may make small but significant contributions to the energy expenditure during exercise. This, however, is a matter of great controversy. Most researchers discount the use of protein as an energy source during physical activity, however substantial current research indicates that protein utilization may increase during prolonged strenuous activity. Recent studies suggested that protein may contribute as much as 5.5 percent of the total energy expenditure during endurance exercise[7] and as much as 10 percent when individuals are carbohydrate depleted.[8] Thus, it appears that for certain activities, such as a marathon, triathlon, or other distance events, protein may be an important, though not a major, energy source for the working muscles. Furthermore, there is no evidence at this time to suggest that increasing protein intake above normal daily requirements will enhance energy efficiency or improve performance.[9,10] Carbohydrates and fats are the muscle's primary fuel sources during exercise and consuming proper amounts of these nutrients is therefore most important in preventing the utilization of large amounts of protein as an energy source during endurance activities.

For some athletes, such as weight lifters and football players, increased muscle bulk is desirable for optimal performance. Many of these athletes therefore believe that high-protein diets and protein supplements are needed during training to augment muscle growth and improve performance. Indeed, protein is needed for muscular development during the conditioning process. In fact, requirements may even be slightly higher during the period when substantial new muscle tissue is being formed.[11] However, protein supplementation above normal dietary intake will not increase muscle tissue growth during training,[9] nor will it enhance physiological work performance.[12] Moreover, excessive protein intake may actually be harmful.

When the body receives more protein than it needs, the liver and kidneys must work harder to metabolize and excrete the nitrogenous protein waste products. The additional burden could be damaging to these organs. Furthermore, the increased fluid excretion associated with the removal of nitrogenous waste products by the kidneys could easily cause an individual to become dehydrated and perform poorly. Such common practices as consuming protein powders or amino acid supplements are therefore contraindicated. Not only are these expensive, but they are unnecessary and potentially dangerous.

The key to increasing muscle size and strength is to eat a well-balanced diet and maintain a regular conditioning program. While training does not require excessive protein intake, it does require extra energy. Therefore, inclusion of adequate calories from carbohydrate and fat is the most important requirement to ensure that dietary protein will be used for the growth and maintenance of muscle cells.

The protein RDA for adults is 0.8g/kg of body weight. Thus a 20-year-old man weighing 154 pounds (70 kg) would require 56 g of protein per day. That is the approximate amount found in 6 ounces of meat, fish, or fowl plus 12 ounces of milk. When one adds together the servings of meats, dairy products, grains, and legumes typically consumed in a day, it is easy to see that the average well-balanced diet supplies more than enough protein. In fact, according to the U.S. dietary guidelines, no more than 12 to 15 percent of the day's calories should come from protein. For athletes with an increased caloric requirement, this could be the equivalent of 1 to 3 g/kg per day, or two to four times the RDA. Such amounts are more than enough to meet both training and competitive needs. Moreover, protein intake in excess of that which can be used for the growth and maintenance of body cells is simply stored as fat, with the remaining nitrogen being excreted in the urine, which can potentiate dehydration and kidney damage.

Vitamins and Minerals

The belief that athletes require more vitamins and minerals than nonathletes is linked to the misconception that these nutrients supply energy. The fact is, vitamins and minerals do not supply energy. They work instead in very minute quantities with enzymes that control the thousands of metabolic reactions that take place in the body each day. Vitamins and minerals aid in the metabolism of carbohydrates, protein, and fats; they help regulate the nervous system; and they are involved in blood clotting and detoxification of alcohol and other poisons. Minerals are also important components of body structure, such as bones and teeth.

Vitamins are classified according to their solubility in fat or water. There are four fat-soluble vitamins—A, D, E, and K—and nine water soluble vitamins—vitamin C, thiamin (B_1), riboflavin (B_2), niacin, folacin, pyridoxine (B_6), B_{12}, pantothenic acid, and biotin.

Minerals are classified as macronutrient elements (calcium, phosphorus, sulfur, sodium, potassium, chlorine, and magnesium) and micronutrient elements, commonly referred to as "trace" minerals (iron, flourine, zinc, copper, iodine, chromium, cobalt, silicon, vanadium, tin, silenium, manganese, nickel, and molybdenum).

Of the vitamins and minerals known to be needed by the athlete, all must be supplied in the diet. Specific allowances have been established for all vitamins and some minerals, including calcium, iron, phosphorus, iodine, magnesium, and zinc. Whether or not these allowances are appropriate for all athletes is currently being debated. Recent studies suggest that extremely active individuals may require more riboflavin, iron, and calcium, depending on the level of exercise and the environmental conditions in which the exercise is performed.[13-16] There is a more detailed discussion of iron and calcium requirements later in this chapter.

Even though some athletes may require more of certain vitamins and minerals, the need for supplementation is usually not necessary if a normal well-balanced diet is consumed. By eating just a few servings from each food group, one can easily obtain and even exceed the RDAs for many vitamins and minerals. Consider, for example, the USRDA for riboflavin (1.7 mg). This is the amount found in a single serving of fortified cereal. The RDA for vitamin C can be satisfied by consuming as little as 5 ounces of orange juice or $\frac{1}{2}$ cup of broccoli.

Though athletes can get all the necessary vitamins and minerals through a normal diet, many still turn to supplementation with the belief that if a little is good, more must be better. They believe that extra vitamins and minerals will improve the functioning of the body during exercise to give them an extra edge over their competitors.

The fact that deficiencies of certain vitamins and minerals can impair performance is well documented; however, numerous investigations have shown that taking excessive or "megadose" vitamin and mineral supplements has no beneficial effect on athletic performance.[17,18] Moreover, athletes who consume large doses of these nutrients may actually be harming themselves.

While most vitamins are well tolerated in amounts that exceed the RDA by two to three times,[19] a higher intake of many may be toxic. The toxicity of fat-soluble vitamins, particularly A and D, has been well established at doses only 10 times higher than the RDA.[20] Excessive intake of water-soluble vitamins, once considered harmless, have also been shown to produce toxicities when ingested in large amounts. Individuals consuming megadoses of B_6, for example, (2 to 6 g per day, or 1,000 to 2,700 times the RDA) have suffered serious neurological impairments and temporary paralysis.[21] Large intakes of vitamin C can cause diarrhea[22] and can interfere with the absorption and metabolism of B_{12}.[20] The ingestion of 3 or more grams of niacin has been shown to interfere with endurance performance by increasing the rate of glycogen use by the muscles and decreasing fatty acid availability during prolonged exercise.[20]

For athletes consuming a normal, well-balanced diet, vitamin supplementation is not only unnecessary, but dangerous. The only time supplementation should be considered is when an athlete habitually omits one of the four major food groups or when a deficiency has been diagnosed clinically. In these cases, individuals should seek the advice of a registered dietitian to determine the type of supplement and proper dosage that will supply the missing or inadequate vitamin or mineral. Ironically, athletes who use supplements are usually those whose diets are adequate, while those athletes with less-than-adequate diets generally do not use supplements.[23] If a vitamin–mineral supplement is warranted, a general multivitamin is usually all that is necessary. However, rather than rely on supplements at all, athletes should be encouraged to obtain all their vitamins and minerals by eating a variety of nutritious foods from the four major food groups.

Iron

Iron is one mineral for which deficiencies are common among athletes, particularly those involved in intense, prolonged physical activity (long-distance runners, triathletes, cross-country skiiers, etc.).[14] Recent studies indicate that iron deficiencies in these individuals may be attributable to inadequate absorption, losses from the gastrointestinal tract, or excessive sweating.[14,15] Inadequate dietary intake is another important factor that contributes to the iron deficiency commonly observed in active athletes.

The RDA for iron is 10 mg/day for men and 18 mg/day for women. Women require more iron than men because of iron losses that occur during menstruation. Few women athletes routinely consume the RDA for this mineral and have a greater incidence of iron deficiency than men.[15,24]

Since iron is necessary for carrying oxygen to the muscles during exercise, iron deficiency would make exercise more difficult by decreasing the amount of oxygen that can be delivered to the working muscles. Extreme fatigue, loss of strength and endurance, and prolonged recovery periods are signs of iron deficiency.

Athletes with a clinically diagnosed iron deficiency usually require supplements to replenish lost stores; however, supplementation should be monitored carefully since extreme iron intakes could be toxic.[19] Moreover, careful selection of iron-rich foods and avoidance of certain dietary factors that decrease iron absorption will help to prevent deficiencies and ensure than requirements are met.

Iron is present in foods in two forms. Heme iron is the most readily absorbed form of iron and is present only in animal tissues, including meat, liver, poultry, and fish. Nonheme iron, also found in animal tissues, accounts for 100 percent of the iron found in vegetable products. Because this form is less well-absorbed, individuals relying mainly on nonheme foods may not be getting all the iron they need. There are, however, certain food components that can influence the absorption of nonheme iron. Enhancers of nonheme iron absorption are vitamin C and a factor present in meat, fish, and poultry. Including a good source of vitamin C, such as a glass of orange juice, a piece of fruit, or a fresh salad, in a meal will help increase the absorption of any nonheme iron present. Having fish or poultry would also augment the availability of iron from grains or vegetables in the same meal.

Another means of obtaining more iron from the diet is to use iron pots and pans, especially when cooking acidic foods. The iron content of spaghetti sauce, for example, increases nearly 3,000 percent (from 3 to 88 mg per $\frac{1}{2}$ cup) when cooked for a few hours in a cast iron pot.[11] Inclusion of "enriched" or "fortified" breads and cereals will also help increase the iron content of the diet since these products have iron added to them.

Two beverages, coffee and tea, have been shown to inhibit substantially the absorption of nonheme iron.[25,26] Athletes wishing to optimize their iron intake would be wise to avoid drinking these beverages or at least refrain from drinking them until after a meal has had some time to digest (from 1 to 2 hours).

The iron content of some foods is listed in Table 5-2.

Calcium

Some athletes, particularly those who tend to restrict caloric intake or limit their consumption of dairy products, are unable to meet their need for calcium through diet alone. Indeed, many elite athletes consume less than 60 percent of the RDA for this important mineral.[23]

The fact that calcium is necessary for the maintenance of strong healthy bones is well known. Less well known is the fact that every day some calcium is removed from the bones to circulate in the blood. Under normal conditions, bone calcium is quickly replaced by calcium from the diet. If, however, dietary calcium intake is low, not all of the bone calcium can be replaced. Prolonged

Table 5-2. Iron Content of Selected Foods

Food	Amount	Iron (mg)	% RDA
Heme sources			
Liver	$3\frac{1}{2}$ oz	9.0	50
Steak, lean	$3\frac{1}{2}$ oz	4.5	25
Hamburger, lean	$3\frac{1}{2}$ oz	4.0	22
Veal	$3\frac{1}{2}$ oz	4.0	22
Lamb	$3\frac{1}{2}$ oz	3.0	17
Turkey, dark meat	$3\frac{1}{2}$ oz	2.5	14
Chicken, dark meat	$3\frac{1}{2}$ oz	2.0	11
Tuna	$3\frac{1}{2}$ oz	2.0	11
Turkey, light meat	$3\frac{1}{2}$ oz	1.0	6
Chicken, light meat	$3\frac{1}{2}$ oz	1.0	6
Fish	$3\frac{1}{2}$ oz	1.0	6
Nonheme sources			
Cold cereals			
Product 19	$\frac{3}{4}$ cup	18.0	100
Total	1 cup	18.0	100
Raisin Bran, Post	$\frac{2}{3}$ cup	9.0	50
Nature Valley Granola	$\frac{2}{3}$ cup	2.0	11
Nutri Grain, Wheat	$\frac{3}{4}$ cup	1.0	6
Hot cereals			
Cream of Wheat, instant	$\frac{3}{4}$ cup	9.0	50
Quaker Instant Oatmeal	$\frac{3}{4}$ cup	7.0	39
Rolled oats, regular	$\frac{3}{4}$ cup	1.0	6
Dried peaches	10 halves	5.0	28
Molasses, blackstrap	2 tbs	5.0	28
Dried figs	10	4.0	22
Baked beans	8 oz	4.0	22
Prune juice	8 oz	3.0	17
Wheat germ	$\frac{1}{4}$ cup	3.0	17
Raisins	$\frac{2}{3}$ cup	2.0	11
Spinach	$\frac{1}{2}$ cup	2.0	11
Tofu	$\frac{1}{2}$ cup	2.0	11
Pasta, enriched	1 cup	2.0	11
Bread, enriched	1 slice	1.0	6
Egg	1 medium	1.0	6

Data from Pennington JT, Church HN: Food Values of Portions Commonly Used. 14th Ed. JB Lippincott, Philadelphia, 1985.

periods of insufficient calcium intake can result in a progressive thinning and weakening of the bones, a painful and debilitating condition known as osteoporosis.

Moderate weight-bearing exercise, such as walking or jogging, seems to offer some protection against bone loss by preserving normal bone mineral content. Thus bones appear denser and stronger in individuals who exercise moderately. In contrast, exteme levels of exercise may have adverse effects on bone density. A recent study demonstrated that many high-mileage female runners with amenorrhea (absence of menstrual periods) had significantly reduced bone mineral content despite adequate dietary calcium intakes.[16] The average bone mineral density of athletes in this study was equivalent to that of a 51-year-old woman. Undoubtedly the problem of bone loss would be compounded in women with low calcium intakes. Thus for female distance runners, calcium requirements may actually be greater than the current RDA of 800 mg/ day. It has been suggested that women younger than 35 years of age should

Table 5-3. Calcium Content of Selected Foods

Food	Amount	Ca (mg)	% RDA
Dairy products			
Yogurt, lowfat	8 oz	415	50
Skim milk	8 oz	302	40
Buttermilk	8 oz	285	35
Swiss cheese	1 oz	272	35
Cheddar cheese	1 oz	204	25
Mozzarella, skim	1 oz	183	25
Ice cream, vanilla	1 cup	176	20
Cottage cheese (1% fat)	1 cup	138	20
Soy milk	8 oz	55	10
Seafood			
Sardines, canned	$3\frac{1}{2}$ oz	372	45
Salmon canned	3 oz	167	20
Oysters, raw	5–8	94	10
Shrimp, raw	$3\frac{1}{2}$ oz	63	10
Vegetables			
Collard greens, cooked	1 cup	304	40
Broccoli, stalk, cooked	3 stalks	264	30
Turnip greens, raw	1 cup	252	30
Beet greens, cooked	1 cup	200	25
Spinach, cooked	1 cup	166	20
Other			
Carob flour	$\frac{1}{2}$ cup	246	30
Molasses, blackstrap	2 tbs	232	30
Tofu	4 oz	145	20
Brewer's yeast	3 tbs	63	10
Corn tortillas	6″ diam	60	10
Almonds	12–15	38	5

Data from Pennington JT, Church HN: Food Values of Portions Commonly Used. 14th Ed. JB Lippincott, Philadelphia, 1985.

be taking in 1,000 mg/day, while those aged 35–50 years may need as much as 1,200 mg/day.

Attention to the calcium content of foods should help individuals to maximize their intake of this vital mineral. Dairy products are the best sources of calcium, but other foods, when selected properly, can contribute appreciable amounts of calcium to the diet. Table 5-3 lists the calcium content of some common foods.

Water

Water is an essential nutrient that comprises as much as 60 percent of an individual's body weight. It is necessary for maintaining blood volume and regulating body temperature through sweating. Athletes engaged in strenuous activity in which sweat production is high have increased requirements for this nutrient.

Some athletes erroneously believe that by restricting water intake during practice the body can be "trained" to reduce its total fluid requirement so that drinking during competition can be minimized. Recent research however, shows that such practices can result in significant impairments in physical performance. In fact, water losses as minimal as 2 percent of body weight (2 to 3 lb) have been shown to reduce physical work performance by as much as 20 percent.[27]

Adequate fluid replacement is therefore critical for optimal sports performance. Unfortunately, the need to replace fluids during training or competition is often underestimated, since losses are not always easy to detect. Water losses can be extreme when individuals exercise in hot, dry, or windy environments. Because sweat evaporates quickly under these conditions, an athlete may not "feel" sweaty. This does not mean that sweat is not being lost. Cyclists, for example, have been known to incur losses up to 5 to 6 L (11 to 13 lb) when racing in the heat. A fully heat-acclimated marathon runner may sweat as much as 9 L in the course of a 3-hour race.[28]

Compounding this water loss problem is the fact that normal thirst is not always a good indicator of how much fluid needs to be replaced. In fact, voluntary fluid replacement during strenuous exercise is at most 50 percent of an individual's actual needs. Thus, without knowing, it is very easy for an athlete to become dehydrated.

The best fluid to ensure against dehydration is plain, cold water. Despite heavy sweat losses, the need for special sport drinks containing electrolytes (i.e., sodium and potassium) is not necessary for the majority of athletes. Although some electrolytes are lost in sweat, the body is never totally depleted. In fact, the relative electrolyte concentration in the body is actually increased during periods of heavy sweating because more water is lost than electrolytes.[6] Thus the need to replace body water is much greater than the need to replace electrolytes. Furthermore, the electrolytes that are lost can easily be replaced by the foods consumed immediately after exercise. Potassium losses, for example, may average 85 mg per pound of sweat.[29] An 8-ounce glass of orange juice (380 mg potassium) or a medium-sized banana (450 mg potassium) can easily replace sweat potassium losses.

Water taken prior to exercise only is not as effective in controlling body temperature as consuming equivalent volumes during the exercise period.[30] Thus water should be taken before, during, and following training or competition. One or 2 cups taken 15 minutes prior to activity followed by 4 to 8 ounces every 10 to 15 minutes is recommended for events that last 30 minutes or longer (e.g., cycling, cross-country skiing, running, vigorous tennis, or football practice). Cold water is preferable because it leaves the stomach faster than warm water and has a cooling effect on the body. For events lasting less than 30 minutes, it is generally not necessary to drink until after the event, since the losses incurred are usually minimal and will not adversely affect performance.

A general rule of thumb to gauge water replacement needs is that for each pound of weight lost during exercise, 2 cups (16 ounces) of water should be consumed. Weight losses in excess of 1 to 2 pounds should signal the athlete that he or she is not drinking enough during the exercise session. Contrary to what many athletes believe, drinking water during activity does not cause muscle cramps. Cramps are the result of serious dehydration and sodium depletion that sometimes occurs in highly trained, heat-acclimated persons who sweat profusely. (Heat-acclimatized individuals can sweat up to twice as much as unacclimatized persons).

Even if heat cramps are a problem, the use of salt tablets to replace sodium losses is not recommended since their ingestion only worsens any existing condition of dehydration or overheating. Salt tablets are highly concentrated substances that, when swallowed, must be diluted with water from the surrounding body tissues before absorption can take place. The obvious consequence is a loss of body water. Salt tablets can also irritate the stomach lining and may cause nausea and vomiting. The suggested treatment for sodium depletion heat cramps is to drink a solution containing $\frac{1}{4}$ teaspoon of salt dissolved in 1 quart of water. Such a solution is much less concentrated and should effectively relieve the cramps, while at the same time ensuring that water is optimally absorbed and replaced. Sodium-depletion heat cramps usually can be prevented altogether by ensuring adequate, but not excessive, dietary sodium intake, which can be accomplished simply by lightly salting foods eaten before and after the exercise session.

NUTRITIONAL STRATEGIES FOR COMPETITION

The consumption of a regular well-balanced diet is relatively more important for overall athletic performance than the food eaten just prior to an isolated competition day. Nevertheless, the food and fluids that are consumed during the several days preceding the event and on the day of the event can have a significant influence on performance.

Precompetition Meals

The purpose of the precompetition meal is not to supply energy for the upcoming event, since this energy comes primarily from the foods consumed during the several days preceding the event. Rather, the preevent meal is necessary to prevent the stored forms of energy from being used prematurely. When food is not provided at regular intervals, the maintenance of normal blood glucose levels occurs at the expense of the body's glycogen stores. Thus if the precompetition meal is skipped, this important energy source becomes compromised even before the start of exercise. While this may not adversely affect athletes involved in short-term events, it can hamper the performance of those engaged in more prolonged endurance events in which the glycogen supply is a major determinant of how long the exercise can be sustained. Another reason for the precompetition meal is that it helps keep individuals from feeling hungry before and during activity.

Food remaining in the stomach during exercise can cause cramps, nausea, and vomiting and can compromise performance by reducing blood flow to the working muscles. To prevent competition between the stomach and muscles for the available blood supply and to avoid gastrointestinal problems, the stom-

Table 5-4. Sample Precompetition Meals

Morning	Afternoon	Evening
Orange juice Plain cereal with fresh fruit (blueberries, raisins, bananas, etc.) Skim milk Whole wheat English muffin with jam or jelly	Sliced turkey breast with lettuce and tomato on wheat bread Fresh fruit salad with low-fat yogurt	Skim milk Tossed salad (lettuce and assorted fresh vegetables) with low-fat dressing Fresh pasta with tomato sauce and light sprinkle of parmesan cheese Whole wheat rolls or bread

ach must be empty at the start of exercise. This can be accomplished by consuming meals that are digested quickly and easily. Foods high in carbohydrate are readily digested and leave the stomach faster than high-fat or high-protein foods, thus the best precompetition meal for all athletes is one that is relatively higher in carbohydrates than protein or fat. Fruits, vegetables, breads, and cereals are therefore good precompetition foods. Some high-protein, low-fat foods, however, such as lean meats and low-fat dairy products, can also be included. Although protein takes longer to digest than carbohydrate, it takes much less time to leave the stomach than fat. Fats in general should be limited during the preevent meal because of their slow digestion and absorption. In addition to carbohydrate-rich foods, every preevent meal should include plenty of water, particularly during hot weather. An additional consideration when planning the preevent meal is portion size. Smaller meals are preferred since they remain in the stomach for shorter periods of time than larger meals.

Ideally, a period of at least 3 to 4 hours is necessary to ensure the complete digestion of a meal. If an individual is nervous before a race, digestion could take even longer because anxiety may reduce the rate of stomach emptying. For some, anxiety may have the opposite effect of enhancing the rate of stomach emptying. In this situation, diarrhea is usually a common problem.

Because liquid foods leave the stomach faster than solid foods, they may be consumed closer to the time of competition, however no foods, even high-carbohydrate foods, should be consumed within 1 hour of competition. Athletes who eat a sweet snack, such as a candy bar or soft drink, as a means of obtaining "quick energy" just before competition or practice may be compromising their performance. Such practices have the effect of lowering blood glucose and accelerating muscle glycogen depletion, which can cause an athlete to become fatigued during the early stages of exercise. In addition, large quantities of concentrated carbohydrates cause fluids to be drawn into the gastrointestinal tract, which precipitates dehydration and increases the possibility of cramping, diarrhea, and nausea.

Included in Table 5-4 are three examples of precompetition meals. Each meal is high in carbohydrate and moderate in protein and contains very little fat.

These recommendations also hold true for meals eaten prior to regular training and practice sessions, but the problems associated with preevent anxiety are usually not so important a factor as they may be prior to competition.

Carbohydrate Loading

The ability to sustain moderate to heavy endurance exercise greatly depends on the initial glycogen content of the muscles and can be enhanced when these levels are elevated. The available evidence suggests that muscle glycogen stores can be maximized by consuming a diet high in carbohydrate for several days preceding the event. This so-called "carbohydrate-loading" technique enables well-trained endurance athletes to increase their muscle glycogen content by as much as two times normal.[6]

The classic carbohydrate regimen consists of three dietary phases, including several days on a low-carbohydrate diet consisting largely of fat and protein during the week before competition followed by carbohydrate loading for several days. During the low-carbohydrate phase, athletes train to exhaustion in an effort to deplete their glycogen stores before the loading phase. While this depletion-loading method has been shown to elevate muscle glycogen content to exceptionally high levels, it also poses several problems for the athlete. Most individuals experience extreme fatigue and irritability in association with the low-carbohydrate phase, which causes them to perform poorly during workouts. Not only is this psychologically detrimental to performance, it could also result in overexertion and injury.[6] In view of these negative factors, it has been recommended that the low-carbohydrate–glycogen depletion phase be eliminated.

Instead, athletes should consume a normal mixed diet (50 percent of calories from carbohydrate) in place of the high-protein–fat phase of the classical regimen and then consume a diet rich in carbohydrates (70 to 80 percent of calories from carbohydrates) in the 48- to 72-hour period prior to the event. This alternative carbohydrate-loading regime has been shown to be as effective in maximizing the muscle glycogen content as the original method, yet is an easier, more comfortable means of obtaining the same results.[6] For nonendurance athletes needing only limited amounts of glycogen during competition, carbohydrate loading is not necessary.

Carbohydrate Intake During Prolonged Exercise

For events lasting 1 to 2 hours, it is generally not necessary to consume additional food during the event. In contrast, during very prolonged, moderate- to heavy-intensity exercise lasting 3 or more hours it becomes important to ingest carbohydrates during the actual event to supplement the body's limited carbohydrate stores.[28] The ingestion of carbohydrate under these conditions enhances endurance and reduces fatigue by slowing the rate of glycogen depletion. This is in marked contrast to carbohydrate ingestion just prior to the start of exercise, which has the opposite effect of facilitating glycogen depletion.

The results of a recent study suggest that solid, rather than liquid, forms of carbohydrate are more effective in reducing the rate of glycogen depletion during prolonged exercise[31]. However, despite this finding, liquid carbohydrates in the form of various sport drinks seem to be preferred since fluid replacement is also essential. Unfortunately, many sport drinks are highly concentrated and may actually limit rather than facilitate fluid replacement. Additionally, athletes may experience abdominal cramps, diarrhea, and nausea following the consumption of drinks with a high sugar content. For optimal absorption and fluid replacement, the carbohydrate concentration of any solution should not exceed 2.5 percent.

Some athletes may argue that a 2.5 percent solution is too weak to make significant contributions to the energy needs during exercise. The fact is, a weak solution provides sugar at a much faster rate than more concentrated drinks that remain in the stomach for longer periods of time. The only time when individuals may elect to consume more concentrated sugar solutions is during prolonged exercise in cold environments, when dehydration and overheating are less of a problem.[6] In this situation, smaller volumes are recommended to ensure optimal stomach emptying.

REFERENCES

1. Smith NJ: Food fraud and the athlete. In Fox EL (ed): Nutrient Utilization During Exercise. Ross Symposium. Ross Laboratories, Columbus, Ohio, 1983
2. Felig P, Wahren J: Fuel homeostasis in exercise. N Engl J Med, 293:1078, 1975
3. Costill DL: Fats and carbohydrates as determinants of athletic performance. In Haskell W, Scala J, Whittam J (eds): Nutrition and Athletic Performance. Bull Publishing, Palo Alto, 1982
4. Costill DL, Sherman WM, Fink WJ et al: The role of dietary carbohydrates in muscle glycogen resynthesis after strenuous running. Am J Clin Nutr, 34:1831, 1981
5. Askew, WE: Fat metabolism in exercise. In Fox EL (ed): Nutrient Utilization During Exercise. Ross Symposium. Ross Laboratories, Columbus, Ohio, 1983
6. Costill DL, Miller JM: Nutrition for endurance sport: carbohydrate and fluid balance. Int J Sports Med, 1:2, 1980
7. Evans WJ, Fischer EC, Hoerr RA, Young VR: Protein metabolism and endurance exercise. Phys Sportsmed, 11:63, 1983
8. Lemon PWR, Mullin JP: Effect of initial muscle glycogen levels on protein catabolism during exercise. J Appl Physiol, 48:624, 1980
9. Wilmore JH, Freund BJ: Nutritional enhancement of athletic performance. Nutr Abst Rev, 54:1, 1984
10. Rasch PJ, Hamby JW, Burns HJ: Protein dietary supplementation and physical performance. Med Sci Sports Exerc, 1:195, 1969
11. Krause MV, Mahan LK: Food, Nutrition and Diet Therapy. 6th Ed. WB Saunders, Philadelphia, 1979
12. Consolazio CF, Johnson HL, Nelson RA et al: Protein metabolism during intensive physical training in the young adult. Am J Clin Nutr, 28:29, 1975
13. Belko AZ, Obarzanck E, Kalwarf F et al: Effects of exercise on riboflavin requirements of young women. Am J Clin Nutr, 37:509, 1983

14. Ehn L, Carlmark B, Hoglund S: Iron status in athletes involved in intense physical activity. Med Sci Sports Exerc, 12:61, 1980

15. Clement D, Taunton J, McKenzie D et al: Iron absorption in iron deficient, enduranced trained females. Med Sci Sports Exerc, 16:164, 1984

16. Drinkwater BL, Nilson K, Chesnut CH et al: Bone mineral content of eumenorrheic athletes. N Engl J Med, 311:277, 1984

17. Grandjean AC: Vitamins, diet, and the athlete. Clin Sports Med, 2:105, 1983

18. Williams MH: Vitamin, iron and calcium supplementation: effect on human physical performance. In Haskell W, Scala J, Whittam J (eds): Nutrition and Athletic Performance. Bull Publishing, Palo Alto, 1982

19. Committee on Dietary Allowance Food and Nutrition Board: Recommended Dietary Allowances. 9th Ed. National Academy Press, Washington, 1980

20. Rudman D, Williams PJ: Megadose vitamins. N Engl J Med, 309:488, 1983

21. Schaumburg H, Kaplan J, Windebank A et al: Sensory neuropathy from pyridoxine abuse. N Engl J Med 309:445, 1983

22. Hoyt CJ: Diarrhea from vitamin C. JAMA, 244:1674, 1980

23. Grandjean AC: Profile of nutritional beliefs and practices of the elite athlete. Paper presented at the LaCrosse Health and Sports Science Symposium, LaCrosse, Wisconsin, 1983

24. Strand SM, Clarke BA, Slavin JL, Kelly JM: Effects of physical training and iron supplementation on iron status of female athletes. Med Sci Sports Exerc, 16:161, 1984

25. Morck TA, Lynch SR, Cook JD: Inhibition of food iron absorption by coffee. Am J Clin Nutr, 37:416, 1983

26. Disler PB, Lynch SR, Charlton RW et al: The effect of tea on iron absorption. Gut, 16:193, 1975

27. Sawka MN, Francesconi RP, Young AJ, Pandolf KB: Influence of hydration level and body fluids on exercise performance in the heat. JAMA, 252:1165, 1984

28. Astrand P, Rodahl K: Textbook of Work Physiology. McGraw–Hill, New York, 1977

29. Costil DL: Dietary potassium and heavy exercise: effects on muscle water and electrolytes. Am J Clin Nutr, 36:266, 1982

30. Gisolfi CV, Copping JR: Thermal effects of prolonged treadmill exercise in the heat. Med Sci Sports, 6:108, 1974

31. Hargraves M, Costill DL, Coggan A et al: Effect of carbohydrate feedings on muscle glycogen utilization and exercise performance. Med Sci Sports Exerc, 16:219, 1981

6 | Mechanics of Injury

Barney F. LeVeau

One of the first things to do when confronting an injured athlete is to determine what is hurt and how the injury occurred. This information can be obtained on the field, in the gymnasium, or in the clinic; it is useful immediately for first aid purposes and later for determining the proper treatment procedure. If the injury is caused by a single event, the athlete often can describe in detail how the injury occurred. If the injury is related to repetitive trauma and overuse, the athlete has greater difficulty describing the mechanism of injury but can tell what movement or activity causes the pain. However, athletes may not know how the injury occurred or may have the wrong idea about how it happened. If the clinician knows the general sequence, then the mechanics of the injury and the amount of damage can be postulated. For example, Gozna emphasized that evaluation of the fracture pattern allows the clinician to determine the mechanism of injury and the amount of energy involved.[1]

The cause, however, must be differentiated from the effect. Understanding the causative force is important. Both O'Donoghue[2] and Slocum[3] stressed the value of accurate evaluation of the injury-producing force. Information about the mechanism of injury is indispensible for several reasons. O'Donoghue and Slocum emphasized the importance of the knowledge of injury mechanics for early detection and prompt diagnosis, both of which are essential for successful treatment of athletic trauma. Prevention of injuries also can be built upon this knowledge.

If the mechanism of injury is established, the clinician can determine more accurately what body parts are injured, what specific tissues may be damaged, and the potential extent of the damage. Hence this knowledge aids in the proper diagnosis and evaluation of the injury.

The plan for treatment of the injured athlete provides for return of the athlete to an uninjured state as soon as possible. Knowledge of how the injury occurred allows the clinician to develop a more efficient treatment plan and to consider treatment for all possible aspects of injury. The type of treatment depends on the causative force. For example, according to Souer, the mechanism of fracture imposes certain rules on the treatment provided.[4] Often an athlete may continue certain parts of training to maintain conditioning or skill without aggravating or involving the injured part. An example of this situation is the overuse injury, calcaneal apophysitis. A young athlete who is running on the junior high track team or playing basketball may be have intense heel pain from running or jumping. A conscientious athlete, however, does not want to stop exercising and lose the conditioning that was gained through vigorous training. Since the clinician knows the mechanism of injury, an alternate exercise regime to maintain cardiovascular conditioning and muscle strength and endurance can be developed. The pull of the gastrocsoleus muscle group enhances the injury. An activity such as riding a stationary bicycle does not overload this muscle group. Thus the athlete can ride a stationary bicycle to maintain conditioning until the injury problem subsides.

Another reason for understanding the mechanisms of injury is injury prevention and control. If it is not known how an injury is caused and how the body reacts to the applied loads, subsequent damage to the body cannot be effectively eliminated or even limited. Knowledge of biomechanical principles applied to the occurrence of injury can help dispel misconceptions about the etiology of athletic injuries. By knowing the specific mechanisms of injury for numerous injuries, the clinician can help develop strategies that will reduce the number and severity of injuries. Although some sports, such as football, rugby, and gymnastics, have inherent risks, these risks can be reduced if the mechanism of injury is understood and corrective means applied. Several means to prevent injuries involving mechanical principles may be employed, including training procedures, rules of the sport, proper coaching techniques, equipment design, and facility construction.

BASIC MECHANICS

The application of force is common to all injuries, from an annoying blister to a crippling fracture. All individuals who work with athletes must understand how the forces involved with each sport may lead to injury. Most musculoskeletal injuries occur in a predictable manner based upon the forces involved and the structure of the region.[1] With sufficient knowledge of biomechanical principles, the structure of the tissue involved, and the reaction of these tissues to the applied forces, the clinician can understand better how to deal with the injury.

Force

Force can be defined as a push or pull, or the entity that tends to cause or modify motion. A force can be described by four important characteristics: point of application, line of application, direction, and magnitude.

The point of application is evident in an injury caused by a direct blow.

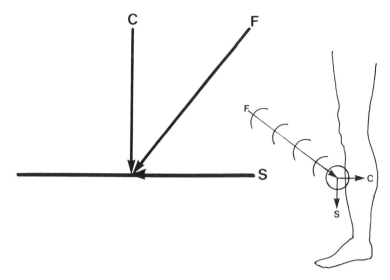

Fig. 6-1.   Line of application of force (F) gives a compression component (c) and a shearing component (S).

The point of application is the location where the applied force and the body part make contact.

The line of application describes the line along which the force is acting. This line passes through the point of application. The angle at which this line approaches the body part determines how much of the force is directed into the body part and how much of the force slides along the surface of the body part (Fig. 6-1). For example, a force more perpendicular (normal force) to a body part may result in a contusion, while a force more parallel to the body part produces an abrasion. A combination of contusion and abrasion occurs if the line lies somewhere between the perpendicular and parallel aspects of the body part.

The direction of the force is represented by an arrowhead on the line of application indicating the vector heading. The direction of the force from an object striking the body is usually obvious. The direction of the force as the body strikes an object is often shown as the reaction force to the body's motion; it occurs in the opposite direction of the motion of the body part (Newton's third law of motion).

The magnitude is the amount of force applied at the point of application. The magnitude of force (F) is often a product of the object's mass (m) and velocity (v) divided by time (t), as derived from Newton's second law of motion:

$$(F = mv/t)$$

This magnitude may be divided into a magnitude that is perpendicular (normal) and one that is parallel to the surface of the body part (tangential).

Load

An external force applied to an object is called a load. The most common loads applied to the body that may produce injury are direct contact with another object, muscle contraction, and inertia of a body part. Bones, ligaments, tendons, muscles, and cartilage provide resisting forces to the applied loads.

Loads from direct contact may be applied anywhere on the body. These forces may produce moments of various magnitudes, depending on where they contact the body.

As muscles attach to bones, they can set up tension upon the apophyses of the bone. They also act singly or in groups to produce tension or compression from their resultant forces or to set up bending moments or torsion.

Inertia is the property of an object to resist the change of motion of an object. This property is the basis of Newton's first law of motion. It acts as a force because it tends to (1) keep an object at rest if the object is stationary, or (2) keep the object moving at a constant velocity (constant speed and straight line motion) unless the object is acted upon by an external force.

Moments

The human body is composed of numerous levers that allow forces to gain a mechanical advantage or provide for increased range of motion. When a load is applied to one arm of the lever, a moment or torque is established so that the lever will tend to turn around a fixed axis. This moment must be resisted by a second moment, which acts in the opposite rotatory direction (Fig. 6-2). The magnitude of each moment (Fxde) depends on the magnitude of the force component (F) perpendicular to the lever arm (moment) and the length of the moment arm (de). The moment arm upon which the load is applied can be called the effort arm. The moment arm of the opposing moment is termed the resistance arm (dr). If the effort arm is greater than the resistance arm, the resisting force (R) must be greater than the load. This relationship generally can be shown by the equation for the second condition of equilibrium ($\Sigma M = 0$), or the sum of the moments acting around an axis equals zero. The relationship of the effort arm (de) to the resistance arm (dr) provides the mechanical advantage (MA) of the lever system:

$$de/dr = MA$$

If the effort arm equals 30 cm and the resistance arm is 5 cm, then the mechanical advantage would be six:

$$30 \text{ cm}/5 \text{ cm} = 6$$

This situation means that six times more force is required by the resisting force than that applied by the load. A long-effort arm may demand that a great amount of resisting force must be available to maintain equilibrium of that particular

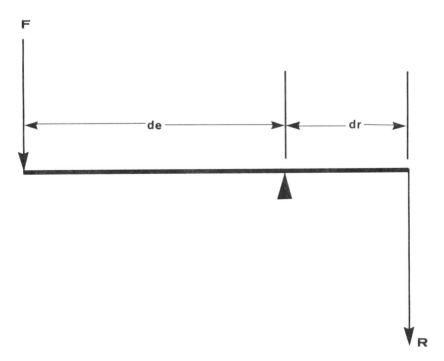

Fig. 6-2.   Lever system with moments F times de and R times dr.

lever system. Force on the tip of a ski and the lever systems in which force is applied to the long limb bones are examples of situations in which the resisting force within the body tissue must be large. Often the body tissue is not sufficiently strong, and injury results.

Stress–Strain

As a load is applied to an object, the object tends to resist any changes in size or shape that may be caused by the load. This resistance or internal reaction to the load is mechanical stress. Stress is measured in units of force per unit area. Stress cannot be determined directly. Stress cannot resist the load completely, so some change in size or shape occurs. This change or deformation is strain. Strain is determined by comparing the change in length with the original length in normal or longitudinal strains and the change in angle with the original angle in shear strain. Strain has no units of measure but can be measured directly. Within limits, the amount of stress may be determined by measuring the strain.

Compression, tension, and shearing are principal types of stresses and strains. Compression occurs when an object has loads acting along the same line in opposite directions to each other. The object decreases in length but becomes greater in perimeter. An example of compression is the loading of an

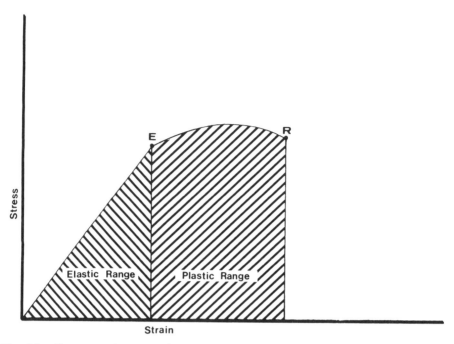

Fig. 6-3.   Stress–strain curve with elastic limit (E) and ruture point (R) showing elastic and plastic ranges.

intervertebral disc. The two surfaces become closer to each other as the sides (annulus fibrosis) bulge out under tension. Tension occurs as loads acting along the same line but in opposite directions lengthen the object. In tension, the object becomes narrower. An example of tension is the loading of a ligament. It can become thinner as it is stretched. Shear takes place as loads acting parallel to each other but in opposite directions create angular deformity of an object. Shearing is present in the intervertebral disc as the fifth lumbar vertebra tends to slide forward on the sacrum.

In many instances, as a load is applied to an object, it immediately deforms. When the load is removed, the object returns to its original size and shape. This reaction is the property of elasticity (Fig. 6-3). Within the range of elasticity, called the elastic range, the amount of strain is directly proportional to the stress (Hooke's law). This ratio of stress to strain represents the stiffness of the material or its ability to resist deformation. This ratio also is called the modulus of elasticity. The larger the ratio or modulus, the less tendency the material has to deform. It is stiffer than a material with a lower ratio value. Bone, for example, has a higher modulus than cartilage. Beyond the elastic limit, the plastic range, Hooke's law no longer holds and strain increases faster than stress. Yield occurs so when the load is removed the material will not return fully to its original size or shape. It maintains a certain amount of deformation. This situation can occur in ligaments that are loaded into the plastic range. If the load is applied continuously to a maximal level, the material will ultimately fail and rupture will result. Torn ligaments and muscles and fractured bones are examples of this phenomenon.

All materials have some degree of elasticity. Some have a property that constitutes resistance to speed of deformation; this is called viscoelasticity. The action of forcing a fluid out of a syringe illustrates this type of resistance. Slow movement requires a greater force. As the load is applied, the developing strain will occur later than the stress. When the load is removed from this type of material, the material remains in the deformed position and does not return to its original size or shape. Most biological tissues have some degree of elastic and viscoelastic properties. The concerted actions of these properties govern the response of the tissue to loading.[5]

The combination of the elastic and viscoelastic properties allows for the response of creep and relaxation of material. Creep occurs when a load is suddenly applied to an object and is sustained for a period of time. The object deforms immediately with the application of the load and then continues to deform gradually. Depending on the magnitude of the load, the deformation may approach a steady state (low load) or progress to a point of rupture (high load). If the load is removed before the point of rupture, the elastic portion of the deformation will be recovered but the viscoelastic deformation will remain. Injury to body tissues may result from prolonged maintenance of a heavy load. Stress relaxation is the response that occurs when a fixed deformation from a load produces a stress. If the amount of deformation remains constant, less load becomes necessary to maintain the deformation and the magnitude of stress within the object will gradually decrease toward zero. Therefore viscoelastic materials respond to a constant load with gradually increasing deformation and to constant deformation with a gradual decreasing of stress.

Energy

Loading an object is also related to work and energy. Energy considerations are very important in injury mechanisms. The source of all injuries seems to be energy exchange: injury occurs when energy from one object is transferred to another object. The total energy involved is the sum of the energy supplied by both objects. The occurrence of an injury depends on the magnitude of the energy, its rate of transfer, its distribution over the various tissues of the body, and the nature of the various body tissues. When the energy present exceeds the ability of the body tissues to absorb and dissipate it, injury results.

Magnitude.   Energy is the ability to do work, and work is produced as a load displaces or moves an object. Work is the product of force times the displacement in the direction of the force. Work is done when an object is lifted above the ground or when an object is deformed. In both situations, potential energy (PE) is developed within the object. The greater the force applied, the greater the resulting energy.

In the first instance (lifting), the object is moved in opposition to the force of gravity. The magnitude of its potential energy equals the product of its mass (m), the acceleration caused by gravity (g), and its height above the ground (h), or

$$PE = mgh$$

When an object falls from a height, the potential energy is gradually changed to kinetic energy (KE). As the object strikes the ground, the potential energy will be zero and the kinetic energy will be maximal. Kinetic energy is related to one-half the mass of the object (m) and the square of its velocity (v), or

$$KE = \tfrac{1}{2}mv^2$$

If an object falls, the kinetic energy at impact equals the potential energy of the object before the fall. A person landing on his or her heel may sustain a fracture of the calcaneus, depending on the height of the fall (mgh) and the ability of the kinetic energy to be absorbed. When two objects collide, the force of the collision is difficult to determine, but the total kinetic energy involved can be calculated based on the kinetic energy ($\tfrac{1}{2}mv^2$) of each of the two objects before the collision and after the collision. In perfectly elastic collisions, the energy after the impact equals the energy before impact. If the energy after is less, then energy was lost in the collision. This energy may be lost by muscle contractions, deformation of tissues, and tearing of tissues. If the energy of impact is too great, injury will occur. Injuries are prevented by covering the area of impact with materials that readily absorb a great amount of energy or disperse the force across a greater area. The force or kinetic energy usually is concentrated at the point of impact. Objects such as mats and pads absorb some energy and dissipate part of the energy to other areas.

In the second situation (work), a force deforms an object. Potential energy is produced within an elastic object as it is deformed. The potential energy, often called strain energy, stored within an elastic object can be calculated by multiplying one-half the force applied (F) times the change in the objects' dimensions:

$$PE = \tfrac{1}{2}Fx\,\Delta d$$

If the deforming force is removed, the energy will be released as kinetic energy. A perfectly elastic object will release the same magnitude of energy as the magnitude of work applied to it. The energy produced up to the elastic limit is recoverable. In most cases, however, some of the energy from the applied work is transferred to heat as the object is deformed or is released as microfractures occur.

The ability of a material to store the energy gained from work done on it and to give back this energy as work when it returns to its original size or shape is called resiliance. Recoverable strain energy comes from elastic materials, such as rubber bands and springs. Resiliance of some materials depends on time. Slow loading and unloading provide sufficient time for some energy to be converted to heat and dissipate into the environment, while rapid loading and unloading tend to return more energy as work. Often a material does not return to its original size and shape at the same rate as it was deformed: some of the energy is dissipated or wasted. This process is called damping. The nature and severity of injuries depends on the magnitude and rate of energy returned from materials, such as a running or playing surface. A strong, stiff surface may give most of the energy back to the body instead of absorbing some of the energy. The greater amount of energy given back to the body can produce injuries.

The work done deforming a material in the elastic range is stored, and much of this energy is returned. Work done deforming an object into the plastic range is not returned. The energy is absorbed, and the object is permanently deformed. For a viscoelastic material, energy is lost at any time during loading and unloading. The energy loss in a viscoelastic material is the process of hysteresis. As a material ruptures, the energy stored as potential energy from the elastic deformation is suddenly released. The energy from work done during plastic deformation has been absorbed and is not released upon failure of the material.

Certain properties of a material can be related to its ability to absorb energy. The ability of a material to absorb energy in the plastic range is its toughness. The area under a stress–strain curve to failure represents the energy absorbed by the material. The more energy the material can absorb before it breaks, the tougher it is. A material that absorbs little energy before it breaks is fragile. A tough material has a greater resistance to fracture than a fragile one.

Another pair of properties relates the amount of strain to energy-absorbing capacity by looking at the magnitude of strain the material allows before it fails. Ductility represents a large amount of nonelastic (plastic) deformation before failure. On the other hand, a brittle material has a small plastic energy-absorbing capacity. High-energy absorption is often related to high ductility. The differentiating point is 5 percent strain. A material that allows greater than 5 percent strain is considered ductile, while a brittle material fails before it deforms by 5 percent. Bone and hard plastics are brittle. Many metals are ductile.

Rate of Applied Energy.   The destruction of tissues during injury depends on not only the magnitude of force but also the rate of force application. The amount of energy a material can store varies with the rate at which it is loaded. The higher the rate of loading, the more energy the material can store before it fails. The higher loading rate increases the stiffness, the ultimate elongation, the strength, and the energy absorption at failure.[1,5] Bone strength with torsion loading increases with the rate of deformation. Its modulus of elasticity increases about 5 percent under faster loading rates.

This ability, however, depends on the type of tissue being loaded. The strength of corticocancellous bone appears to increase more rapidly than ligament strength as the rate of loading is increased. For example, an avulsion fracture may occur as a bone–ligament is loaded slowly under tension. At a faster loading rate, the bone does not pull loose but the ligament tears. The rate of loading also affects the amount of damage that can occur with injury. When a material fails (breaks), energy is released. The faster-loaded material will gain more energy. Therefore, upon failure, more energy will be released. The rate of loading influences the pattern of fracture and the amount of soft tissue damage occurring with the fracture. With a low rate of load application only a single crack occurs, accompanied by little displacement or soft tissue damage. At higher loading rates, the fracture becomes comminuted and the amount of soft tissue injury increases. Thus the greater the energy to produce a fracture, the more complex the fracture pattern.

Absorption of Energy. The distribution of energy affects the type of damage that may occur. As work is done on a body area, energy is developed in several areas. For example, as a body lands on the ground, elastic deformation takes place in the bones, ligaments, tendons, muscles, and ground. Depending on the magnitude of the load and the rate of loading, plastic deformation may occur in these materials. One or more of these tissues may fail if the load is too great.

The contraction of muscles can be an important factor in absorbing energy for the prevention of injury. The muscles can absorb a great amount of energy as they allow for controlled movement of the joints of the body. For example, a person landing on his or her feet does not allow his or her muscles to absorb much of the energy unless the knees and hips can begin to flex at impact. Without this flexion, the bones, cartilage, and ligaments must take a greater and faster load. On the other hand, if the athlete is taught to roll or is allowed to slide as he or she falls, the energy is absorbed over a larger area of the body during a longer period of time.

The type of ground covering may also have a great effect on the energy absorption of the body. A stiff, resilient material will give the energy back to the body, while a less resilient viscoelastic material will absorb some of the energy so that the body will have less energy to distribute and absorb. The differences in hardwood floor, cement, artificial turf, grass, asphalt, and brand name coverings should be considered for the prevention of injury, while maintaining the integrity of the activity. Jumping pits are a good example of this concept: the old sawdust and sandpits have given way to sponge and air bags for greater energy absorption, allowing the jumper or vaulter to increase the magnitude of the jump without having as great a chance for injury. Various pads and cushions in equipment designed for protection of the individual must be based on the ability of the material to spread out and absorb much of the energy before it is applied to the body.

Nature of Body Tissues

The physical properties of the various body tissues affect how easily they may be damaged. Research concerning these properties has been extensive, but most has been on nonliving or animal tissue. The results have varied considerably, but some general traits are presented below.

Mature bone seems to fail near its limit of elasticity. This means that bone has very small plastic range and therefore is considered brittle. Bone tends to be viscoelastic in nature, but it is dominated by elastic properties. As the loading rate increases, however, bone reacts in a more viscoelastic manner. Bone provides greatest resistance to compression (15,000 psi) and is weakest with shear stress (8,000 psi). Tension (12,000 psi) resists less load than compression but more than shear.[6] The fibers of bone are arranged so that the mechanical properties vary with the direction of loading. Longitudinal loading of bone results in different behavior than transverse loading. In general, bone will strain 1 to 4 percent before it fails. More specifically, cortical bone fractures at about 2 percent strain, while trabecular bone fractures at about 7 percent strain. Trabecular bone has a higher energy storage capacity than cortical bone.[7] Cortical bone has a greater modulus of elasticity than trabecular bone; hence it is stiffer by 10 to 20 times. Age also affects the properties of bone. Younger bone is more elastic than mature bone. As mature bone ages, it decreases in strength and strain to failure and increases in brittleness.[5]

Soft tissues of the musculoskeletal system vary somewhat in their structure and mechanical properties. Tendons, ligaments, and cartilage contain a large percentage of collagen fibers and a variable but generally small percent of elastin fibers. Collagen fibers in soft tissue are in a wavy configuration when they are not under tension. As a tension load is applied, the fibers become straightened. During this time, stress is low compared with strain. After the fibers have been straightened, they become stiff. Collagen fibers fail at about 6 to 10 percent strain[5,7] and are about 50 percent as strong as bone.[7] They show considerable hyteresis in the elastic range and undergo considerable plastic behavior near the breaking point; therefore they can absorb energy without returning it to the loading process. Elastin fibers, in contrast, fail just beyond 200 percent strain. They produce very little resistance as stress until about 200 percent strain,[5,7] when they become very stiff, offer a relatively great amount of stress, and rupture as if they were brittle. They have a much lower modulus of elasticity and are less viscoelastic than collagen fibers. They have about 10 percent of the strength of bone.[7]

Tendons are composed of mostly collagen fibers, which are aligned in a parallel fashion to resist high tensile loads. The modulus of elasticity of a tendon is about 5 to 10 percent that of bone.[5] Its tensile strength is about 70 percent that of cortical bone.[5] Ligaments have mostly a parallel fiber arrangement but also have some nonparallel fibers, most of which are collagen. They have, however, more elastic fibers than tendons so that they have less loss of energy to heat in the elastic range. Both ligaments and tendons increase in strength and stiffness as the rate of loading increases. They both demonstrate creep and stress relaxation.

Cartilage is loaded mainly in compression, but its fibers are under constant tension because of its high water content. Its modulus of elasticity is about 0.1 percent that of cortical bone. Its tensile strength is about 4 to 5 percent that of cortical bone. Although cartilage is highly viscoelastic, at a high rate of

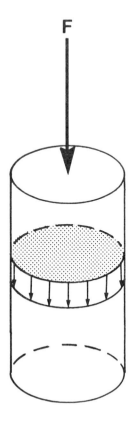

Fig. 6-4.   Compression from uniaxial loading.

loading it is more elastic in character than at low loading rates. Cartilage also exhibits creep and relaxation.[5]

TYPES OF LOADING

Stress is generally developed in objects by three different types of loading: uniaxial, bending, and torsion. Bending and torsion are the result of loads acting at a distance from a relative fixed axis. Bending and torsion, therefore, are caused by moments.

Uniaxial

The uniaxial load on a cylindrical object is located over the exact center of the cylinder in line with the axis of the cylinder (Fig. 6-4). Ideally, the load is applied perpendicular (normal) to the surface of the object with no moments established within the object. Uniaxial loading tends to generate stress evenly throughout the material. Regardless of whether the load is applied at one point or over the entire surface, the resulting stress is uniform throughout the object.

If the load is tensile, the object becomes longer but also more narrow as it demonstrates compression strain as well. This situation decreases the cross-sectional area of the object and therefore increases the stress within the object. Shear stresses and strains at one-half the magnitude of the maximal tension occur at 45 degrees with the direction of the tension load. If the load is compressive, the object will be shorter, but it will exhibit tensile strain and become wider. This change in width sets up shearing stresses and strains at 45 degree angles with the line of compression loading and at one-half the compression magnitude.

Bending

Bending is often illustrated by a horizontal beam. The load may be either at one point or distributed in some manner along the beam. For simple or cantilever bending, the beam is fixed at one end while the bending load is applied at the other (Fig. 6-5). This type of bending is evident as a diver stands on the end of a diving board. Free bending occurs in a beam that is supported at both ends with the bending load applied somewhere between the two supports (Fig. 6-5B). If one point load is applied, this bending may be referred to as three-point bending. A person sitting in the middle of a simple bench is an example of this bending situation. In either simple or free bending, as the beam bends from the load, one surface becomes convex (tension strain) and the other becomes concave (compression strain). Tension stress is developed within the convex side, while compression stress is established in the concave side. These stresses are maximum at the surfaces of the beam and decrease toward the center. A neutral plane with no longitudinal strain occurs at the center of the beam where a transition of tension stress is produced within the deformed beam. Horizontal shear is perpendicular to the applied load. Horizontal shear is maximal at the neutral plane and decreases to zero at the surface of the beam. Horizontal shear can be illustrated by bending a ream of paper or a stack of flat lumber. Vertical shear develops across the beam parallel to the load and supporting force. The bending moment applied to the simple beam is a product of the load and the distance to the point of loading. As a bending moment is applied to the beam, a resisting moment is established within the beam to resist the deformation. The magnitude of the resistance is in reaction to the bending moment. The resisting moment, however, cannot exceed a specific value based upon the thickness of the beam, the type of material of which the beam is composed, and the area moment of inertia of the beam. If the limit of the resisting moment is exceeded, the beam will break. This failure of the beam initially occurs in the area of the greatest tension strain. A greenstick fracture is an example of this type of failure.

The thickness of the beam has a great effect on its ability to resist bending. The resisting effect is related to the cube of the thickness. If the thickness is doubled, the resisting effect is increased by 8. If the thickness is quadrupled, the resistance increases by 64 times. Therefore a bone of greater thickness provides greater resistance to fracture. The composition of the object being

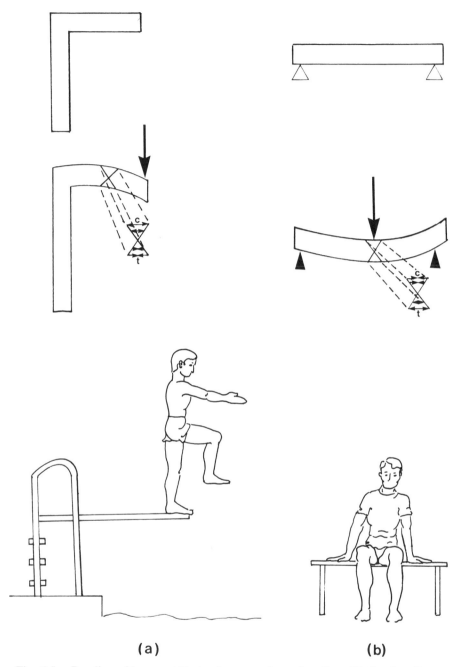

Fig. 6-5. Bending of beams: (A) simple or cantilever bending (B) free bending.

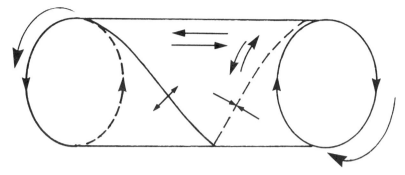

Fig. 6-6. Loading a rod in torsion.

bent is also important. For example, bone is stronger than cement but weaker than steel in bending. The area moment of inertia is another factor that affects the resistance of an object to bending. This property of the material is based on its shape. The further the material of the object is distributed from the neutral plane, the greater its resistance to bending. There is a different formula for area moment of inertia for each type of cross section. A solid cylindrical rod is less rigid than other shapes. A rectangular beam of the same type and same amount of material will resist bending in the thicker dimension better than the rod, but will have less resistance if the load is applied in the direction of the lesser thickness. For example, in a rectangular beam, the bending resistance to a load applied in the thicker dimension can be 16 times greater than the bending resistance to a load applied in the thinner dimension. A similar situation exists in the I-beam. A hollow cylinder composed of the same type and amount of material has five times greater bending resistance than a solid cylindrical rod, greater than the maximum bending resistance of the solid rectangular beam, and slightly less than the maximum bending resistance of the I-beam. The hollow cylinder, however, provides the same resistance in all directions. Therefore the design of long bones provides an efficient resistance to bending in all directions.[1,6,7]

The ability of an object to resist a load in bending also depends on the length of the beam. The greater the distance of the load from a fixed point of the beam, the greater the beam will bend. This change in bending resistance is inversely proportional to the cube of the length. Tripling the length of the beam will decrease its bending resistance by 27 times.[5]

Torsion

Torsion is often illustrated with a cylindrical rod. Torsion occurs when moments are applied to the rod so that it twists around its axis (Fig. 6-6). The moments are maximum at the outer surface and decrease to zero at the rod's neutral axis. The two ends of the object rotate in opposite directions, producing compression, tension, and shear stresses. Maximal compression and tension

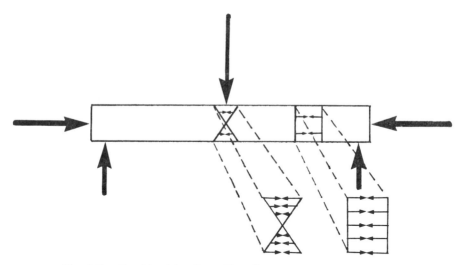

Fig. 6-7. Combined loading of bending and axial compression.

stresses are developed at a 45-degree angle to the axis of the moments. Maximum shear occurs parallel and perpendicular to the neutral axis of the rod. The magnitude of shear stress is the greatest at the surface of the rod. These stresses provide a resisting moment that tends to resist torsional deformation. The resisting moment, similar to bending, depends on the radius of the object, the type of material of which the object is composed, and the polar moment of inertia of the object. An object with a greater radius can resist a greater torque load. The resistance to torsion is increased by the 4th power so that doubling the radius of an object increases its resistance by 16 times.

The shape of the cross section of the object affects the resistance to torsion. Each shape of cross section has a different formula for polar moment of inertia. The hollow cylindrical shape of bone provides greater resistance to torsion than the same amount of material in a solid cylinder shape. The upper tibia, for example, has a larger radius and relatively more bone located near its circumference than the distal end of the tibia. This is why the distal tibia fails more often than the proximal tibia. The major failure follows the strain line of tension. This is illustrated by the spinal fracture of a long bone.

The ability of an object to resist a load in torsion also depends on the length of the rod. The longer the rod with a greater distance between the moments causing torsion, the less its resistance to torsion. The change in torsional stress is inversely proportional to the length of the rod.

Combinations of Loading

If a beam is loaded by axial compression while it is bent, the stresses within the beam will be modified (Fig. 6-7). The bending beam has compression on the concave side and tension on the convex side. The additional compression

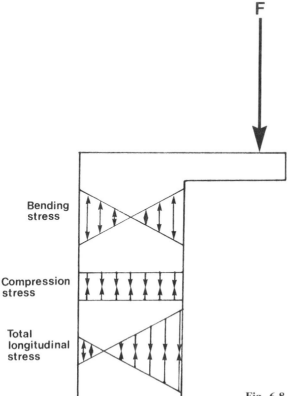

F

Bending
stress

Compression
stress

Total
longitudinal
stress

Fig. 6-8. Eccentrically loaded column.

stress on the concave side decreases the tension stress on the convex side and moves the neutral plane toward the convex side. The axial force, if great enough, can eliminate the tension stress completely from the beam. Several examples of this situation occur in the body. The most common axial force applied to the long bones as beams is muscle force. Muscle force, then, can control the magnitude of compression and tension within the shaft of the bone. Body weight on the head of the femur sets up compression and tension within the femoral neck by cantilever bending. Loading by the hip abductor muscles provides a force component of axial compression, which reduces the magnitude of tension within the superior aspect of the femoral neck.

An eccentrically loaded column combines the effects of compression and bending similar to the uniaxial and bending combination. A column is a relatively slender weight-supporting structure generally in the vertical position. The loading is parallel to the axis, as in uniaxial loading. The load, however, is not in line with the axis of the column. This off-center, or eccentric, loading provides the same magnitude of compression as if the load were uniaxial, but it also produces a moment that tends to bend the column (Fig. 6-8). The distance of the load from the axis of the column times the magnitude of the load determines the magnitude of the bending moment. A resisting moment is established within the column. Compression is on the same side as the off-centered load, while tension is developed on the opposite side. The compression from the axially directed load will be added to the stresses from the resisting moment. The compression on the load side will be increased and the tension on the opposite side will be decreased. The neutral plane will be moved away from the load. An example of eccentric column loading is stress in the lower limbs during standing or the stress in the upper limb as one pushes his or her hand against a heavy door. Several other combinations of loading bones have been discussed in detail.[8-10]

CATEGORIES OF INJURIES

Certain conditions always must be considered when determining how an injury occurred and what tissues may be damaged. These include the type of load applied; the position of the body part; the characteristic of the load, including the point of application, line of application, direction, and magnitude; and the resistance of the body structure. Damage may occur directly at the point of application or at a distance from the load application. This response is established by lever systems and by transfer of energy directly from one tissue to another.

In general, injuries can be divided into two major categories: traumatic disruptions and overuse syndromes. These categories also can be separated into macrotrauma with sudden injury and microtrauma with insidious onset. A distinguishing feature between traumatic disruptions and overuse syndrome seems to be the magnitude of force involved. A greater load gives immediate trauma. With lesser load, failure takes longer to occur.

Traumatic Disruptions

Traumatic disruptions can be considered an immediate result of direct loading to the area. The tissues are damaged when rapidly applied loads produce strain beyond which tissues can tolerate. The loads may be applied uniaxially by compression or tension, by bending, by torsion, or by a combination of loading types. The loads may come from contact or noncontact. Most athletic injuries are caused by contact forces. The force is delivered in some manner to a certain part of the body and the kinetic energy is transmitted to various body structures according to the characteristics of the force applied. Contact may occur between participants or between an object and participant. Some injuries can occur from noncontact. These injuries are self-induced and often arise from the athlete producing force or movements that the body tissues cannot withstand.

Contact Injuries

Types of injuries resulting from direct contact to an area include contusions, open wounds, fractures, dislocations, and concussions. Any area of the body is vulnerable to a single, direct blow. Contusions often occur to muscles such as the quadriceps as an opponent's knee drives into the athlete's thigh. They occur to the iliac crest and greater trochanter as an athlete lands on a hard surface, such as artificial turf or gymnasium floor. Contusions to the kidneys or spleen may follow a blow to the abdominal area by a helmet or baseball. Contusions are a major result of compression to an area. Lacerations follow a direct blow by a sharp object, such as a hockey puck or lacrosse stick. They may also result from contact that stretches the skin apart, such as a fall on the elbow or knee. Baseball cleats can slice into the skin. Tension and shear loads to the skin produce most lacerations. Abrasions occur from shearing as the skin is scraped across a surface. Often abrasions result on a track, the gymnasium floor, or artificial turf as the athlete is moving rapidly, falls, and slides along the surface. Abrasions also may be produced by improperly fitting equipment that rubs the skin. Puncture wounds are less common than lacerations or abrasions but may occur in activities such as track and field that include sharp, pointed equipment. Fractures from direct contact may follow a fall, contact with an implement, contact with part of the facility, or contact with another athlete. The face, ribs, patella, skull, and long bones are vulnerable to force sufficient to cause breaking of the bones.

Dislocations result from direct contact during falls or collisions with another object or person. Acromioclavicular dislocations (separation) and elbow dislocations may be produced as the athlete lands directly on the tip of the shoulder or on the elbow. Lateral force applied to the patella may cause it to sublux or dislocate. Shearing or tension stresses are established as these contact forces arise. Fracture of the skull may follow direct contact to the head. Brain damage, however, may occur without any evidence of skull fracture. Inertia is evident in concussions. The brain can move inside the cranial vault. If a rapidly moving head is suddenly stopped by contact, the brain may keep moving. Compression of the brain will occur at the side of the direction of motion; tearing of the tissue from tension failure will occur on the opposite side. This type of injury also may be created by an outside force that strikes the head, causing the skull to move as the brain tends to remain stationary. In this instance, the compression will occur on the side of contact and tearing on the opposite side.

The occurrence of injuries by direct contact to an area often depends on the nature of the activity and protective measures taken. Activities that cannot be performed without some chance of contact with an object, whether it is another participant, a piece of equipment, or part of the facility, must allow for protection of the athlete. This protection comes in the form of materials that disperse the force over a large area, often covering other materials, that absorb a large amount of the contact energy. Football pads are a good example of an initial hard surface that spreads the load over soft material that absorbs the energy. A catcher's mask is another example. If the athlete will be colliding with an object, the energy-absorbing material should be placed so that it will make the initial contact. Energy-absorbing material around basket supports and along walls near a playing area provide some protection. The hard shell of a football helmet does not, because the helmet often can be used as a weapon to injure an opponent.

The major injury may not always occur at the point of application of the load: the energy from the contact may be transferred to another part of the body through body tissues, or the force may be transferred to another area by the lever systems of the skeleton. These transfer mechanisms may combine to cause the resulting injury. One example of these mechanisms in action is the variety of injuries that may follow as an individual falls on an outstretched hand. The position of each segment of the upper limb and the position of the body determine the type of loading in each area and the response of the tissue to the loading. The tissues in the weakest area, or the area that is loaded the most, will fail first.

Forced hyperextension (dorsiflexion) of the wrist sets up a moment through the metacarpals that produces a pinching action on the navicular bone. A fractured navicular may result. The dorsally placed forces may proceed proximally and produce a combination of impaction and shearing at the distal ulnar epiphyseal plate. The ulnar styloid may be fractured. Wrist hyperextension with forearm supination allows for shearing and compression on the radial side of the forearm. Fracture of the radial styloid or posterior displacement of the distal radial epiphysis may occur.

The energy from the fall may continue up the forearm. The two bones may become bent and break in a greenstick fracture. Additional axial loading may cause compression, or a torus fracture. If the hand becomes fixed to the ground and an external rotational force causes torsion of the humerus and ulna, the ulna may break, followed by dislocation or fracture of the radius.

The most common position of the elbow during a fall on the outstretched hand is abduction combined with hyperextension. In this position, the force is transmitted along the radius and some of the energy is absorbed by the interosseous tissue and muscles. A valgus force sets up compression on the radial side and tension on the ulnar side of the elbow area. The loading type is a combination of uniaxial and bending. The head or neck of the radius or capitellum of the humerous may be fractured from compression between the capitellum and radial head. Avulsion of the medial epicondyle or tearing of the medial collateral ligament may result. If the elbow is held firmly in extension, an oblique fracture of the olecranon may occur. With the force directed through the ulna on a supinated forearm, an extended or partially extended elbow may dislocate posteriorly. Fracture of the humerus can take place in the proximal end if it is abducted, extended, and externally rotated, and in the shaft if the arm twists during the fall.

If the force reaches the shoulder area, four common injuries may occur. The rotator cuff muscles may be compressed between the humeral head and the coracoacromial ligament or acromian, or the acromioclavicular joint may be subluxed if the arm is in the abducted position. Partial abduction of the arm sends the force to fracture the clavicle. If the arm is fully abducted, the glenohumeral joint may be subluxed or dislocated.

Injuries to the ankle are caused mainly by contact forces applied at a distance from the joint with the foot being forced into eversion, plantar flexion, dorsiflexion, or external rotation. The most important aspects for ankle injuries are the position of the foot at impact and the direction of the contact force. The following foot positions and force directions lead to the most common injuries. With the foot in supination and inversion, a load from the lateral side of the foot places the lateral ligaments on tension. Rupture of these ligaments and/or avulsion of the distal fibula may occur. If the load is of sufficient magnitude or sufficient duration, the distal end of the tibia may be fractured by bending and shear. Anterior ligaments are torn and the metaphysis of the tibia may be fractured if the load is directed posteriorly with the foot supinated and plantar flexed. External rotation of the foot while it is supinated or pronated and everted results in a spiral fracture of the distal tibia and transverse or oblique fracture of the fibula. A load to the abducted and everted foot from the medial side may result in torn deltoid ligaments or avulsed distal tibia from tension and a fractured distal fibula from shearing and bending as it is struck by the talus and calcaneus.

The knee is one of the most frequently injured areas. The most common mechanism of injury is force from the lateral side of the fixed lower limb with combined uniaxial, bending, and external torsion loading. The result is tear of the medial collateral and anterior curciate ligaments, the posterior capsule, and the medial meniscus. Fracture of the femoral physis on the medial side may accompany these damaged tissues. Similar bending and torsional stresses are established as a soccer player strikes a ball and opponent with a vigorous adduction–flexion motion at the hip.

Several other traumatic injuries are caused by contact forces. A few examples follow. Forces from uniaxial loading cause compression fractures. Shock waves to the spine from bouncing on a snowmobile seat or landing on extended lower limbs can fracture the vertebral body or herniate a disc. Compression fractures of femoral condyles, tibial condyles, and distal tibia can follow loads applied uniaxially to the lower limbs. Injuries to the fingers are often caused by bending moments. A ball may strike the athlete's thumb and tear the collateral ligament of the metacarpophalangeal joint (gamekeeper's thumb) or fracture the base of the thumb. The end of an extended finger may be flexed forcibly from catching a ball or striking an object. A torsion load to the leg results in a spiral fracture of the tibia as the tip of a ski strikes an object. In general, uniaxial loading produces compression fractures, bending causes torn ligaments and transverse fractures, and torsion loads lead to spiral fractures.

Noncontact Injuries

Traumatic injuries arise from forces other than contact. Muscular contractions and inertia also can cause severe injuries. Rapid contractions of the muscles with the resistance from body weight, combined with force of some other objects, produce a great tension load on the tendon–bone interface. Avulsion fractures result in areas such as the ischial apophysis, pubic tubercle, lesser trochanter, anterior–superior iliac spine, anterior–inferior iliac spine, infrapallar pole, and tibial tuberosity. A spiral fracture of the humerus resisted by the inertia of the forearm and missile establish torsion within the humerus. If the loads are great enough, fracture will result. Muscle strains may result from strong muscle contraction. Tearing of the quadriceps muscles may be produced by sprinting. As the quadriceps muscles contract to swing the leg through rapidly, the inertial resistance of the leg may be sufficient to rupture some muscle fibers, especially if the muscles are fatigued. Once the leg is moving rapidly during the swing phase of running, it must be stopped before foot strike. The inertia of the moving leg requires considerable muscle force by the hamstring muscles, and tearing of fibers of the hamstring muscles result. A similar situation takes place during the throwing action, because the external rotators of the humerus tend to decelerate the moving arm. Inertia may cause acceleration and deceleration injuries to the cervicle spine. Acute flexion of the area may cause a fracture of the vertebral body. Hyperextension may produce fracture of the pedicle, lamina, or spinous process. Avulsion of the anterior longitudinal ligament also may occur. The fractures will be accompanied by soft tissue injuries to the area.

Overuse Syndromes

Overuse syndromes are the result of chronic cyclic activity. They can be produced by low repetition of high-magnitude loads or high repetition of normal loads. The term "fatigue" is used to denote failure of a material by repeated loading and unloading of a magnitude within the stress limits of the material. The load is below the breaking point of the tissue and may be within the elastic range. The lower the load, the greater the number of cycles needed to produce failure of the tissue. For most tissues, a load limit exists below which an infinite number of cycles will not cause failure. A common factor for all repetitive loading types is that microtrauma occurs repeatedly. Overuse injuries can be related to increased intensity of activity in several ways. They may be a result of excessive repetition with normal anatomy; high repetitions with anatomical malalignment or imbalances; improper training techniques; or improper equipment or facilities, such as footwear or playing surfaces. The lesions can involve tendons, tendon and bone junctions, bone, and ligaments. Most often the loads come from tension, compression, and bending. Tension stresses are set up in apophyses of a bone as the tendon–bone interface is chronically loaded. If the loading is too great, failure will result. Several examples of this type of chronic injury exist in athletic activities. Medial epicondylar epiphysitis (Little League elbow) develops from the extreme valgus stress motion. The strong internal rotators, horizontal adductor and extensor muscles of the shoulder, and trunk motion bring the humerus forward rapidly. The inertia of the forearm, hand, and ball moving initially backward resist the violent change of direction and acceleration. The combined forces place tension on the medial side and compression on the lateral aspect of the elbow. At the same time, vigorous contraction of the flexor–pronator muscles of the forearm add to the tension on the medial epicondyle. With repeated motion, the medial epicondyle becomes avulsed. Osteochondritis from the repeated compression may take place at the capitellum or head of the radius. A similar condition exists as an athlete swings a racket from the backhand position. In this situation, the lateral side of the elbow is stressed in tension. The wrist extensor muscles pull on the lateral epicondyl of the humerus (tennis elbow).

Running and jumping create repetitive muscle contractions that place tension on the muscle attachments of the lower limbs. Painful syndromes result, most commonly apophysitis of the tibial tuberosity (Osgood–Schlatter Disease) or inferior pole of the patella (Sinding–Larsen–Johannsson syndrome), and calcaneal apophysitis (Sever's disease). Strong, repetitive loading of these areas may cause tension failure in the tendon–bone interface.

Traction at the sites of the anterior and posterior tibialis muscle attachment may produce pain. This tension load causes shin splints. Another major incapacitating overuse tension injury is plantar faciitis. Repetitive tension on the plantar fascia is brought about by the cyclic loading of the calcaneus and metatarsal heads. Pain and inflammation often occur at the fascial–bone interface.

Repetitive compression loading produces several examples of overuse syndromes. Constant pounding of the calcaneus can lead to contusion of the heel (jogger's heel). Proper footware, which absorbs the energy from the pounding, can prevent this problem. Growth reactions to compression loading ultimately may lead to degenerative joint problems. Chronic loading of the joints may cause microfactures of the trabeculae followed by bone remodeling and stiffening of the subchondral bone. Common areas of this problem are the ankle, elbow, knee, hip, and intervertebral joints. One of the most common overuse problems is repetitive stress syndrome, which seems to occur secondary to combined compression and shearing (friction) loading. Insufficient loading on one side and overloading on the other side of the posterior patellar surface may cause the growth reactions of softening, fibrillation, and erosion of the patella cartilage. Compression with rubbing also creates annoying conditions, such as iliotibial band syndrome, when the iliotibial tract rubs across the femoral condyle or across the greater trochanter.

Examples of other overuse syndromes are swimmer's shoulder, breast stroker's knee, Little League shoulder, and spondylolisthesis. These conditions are caused by repetitive loads acting at a distance from the damaged area. Bending moments and torsion loading magnify the forces to the localized tissues, which often fail in tension.

Stress fractures are one of the more common overuse injuries. They may be related to abnormal loading applied to normal bone (fatigue fracture) or to normal loading of a bone that is deficient in elastic resistance (insufficiency fracture). Energy absorption in the environment can be a major contributing cause. For example, if the running surface is too hard, it will not absorb the body's energy but will return it to the body. Shoes that are not built of energy-absorbing materials will allow the energy to be passed on to the foot. Muscles will help absorb some of this energy, but as they become fatigued they will absorb less energy. This, in turn, requires other soft tissues and bones to absorb the energy. In the bones such as the metatarsals and fibula, the loading type is that of a bending beam with cyclic patterns of tension and compression. This process brings about a series of steps that may result in fracture. The process begins with excessive elastic deformation, followed by recoil of the bone. The circumferential lamelae become unravelled and local bone resorption begins. Resorption of bone is followed by replacement with osteonal bone. In this remodeling activity, bone resorption progresses faster than bone formation. The bone therefore becomes weaker, providing a greater chance for small fractures to occur. Continued loading may cause more complicated fractures. Common sites of stress fractures are the metatarsals, tibia, fibula, calcaneus, and the pars interarticularis of the vertebra.

SUMMARY

Most injuries to athletes involve the musculoskeletal system. The type of injury depends on several factors: the type of load, the ability of a material to resist a load, the magnitude of the load, the rate of loading, the distribution of the energy, certain properties of the tissues, and the type of loading. These factors are based on the ideal mechanical situation. The human body, however, is not ideal mechanically. The strength of the tissues varies in different loading situations; the bones are not shaped like perfect cylinders; the body tends to repair itself; each athlete is different in size and skill; and each loading situation is not exactly the same.

Injuries are often explained by materials of the body and their ability to absorb or dissipate kinetic energy. The energy that produces injuries is dissipated in several ways: some is lost as the tissue is permanently deformed, some is lost as the intermolecular bonds break apart (fracture), some is lost in motion of the tissue fragments, and some is lost as it is dissipated to surrounding tissues. By identifying injuries in a mechanical context, clinicians can develop better clinical understanding of the injurious events and techniques for diagnosis, treatment, and prevention.

REFERENCES

1. Gozna ER: Biomechanics of long bone injuries. p. 1. In Gozna ER (ed): Biomechanics of Musculoskeletal Injury. Williams and Wilkins, Baltimore, 1982
2. O'Donoghue DH: Injuries to the knee. Am J Surg 98:463, 1959
3. Slocum DB: The mechanism of football injuries. JAMA 170:1640, 1959
4. Souer R: Fractures of the Limbs: The Relationship between Mechanism and Treatment. La Clinique Orthopedique, Brussels, 1981
5. Cochrane GVB: A Primer of Orthopaedic Biomechanics. Churchill Livingstone, New York, 1982

6. Frost HM: Orthopedic Biomechanics. Charles C. Thomas, Springfield, Ill., 1973
7. Frankel VH, Nordin M: Basic Biomechanics of the Skeletal System. Lea and Febiger, Philadelphia, 1980
8. Dumbleton JH, Black J: An Introduction to Orthopedic Materials. Chalres C. Thomas, Springfield, Ill., 1975
9. Ogden JA: Skeletal Injury in the Child. Lea and Febiger, Philadelphia, 1982
10. Alms M: Fracture mechanics. J Bone Joint Surg 43B:162, 1961

SUGGESTED READINGS

Adams JE: Injury to the throwing arm: a study of traumatic changes in the elbow joints of boy baseball players. Calif Med 102:127, 1965

Adams JE: Little league shoulder: osteochondrosis of the proximal humeral epiphysis in boy baseball pitchers. Calif Med 105:22, 1966

Adams JE: Bone injuries in very young athletes. Clin Orthop 58:129, 1968

Atwater A: Biomechanics of overarm throwing. Exerc Sports Sci Rev 7:43, 1979

Bateman JE: Cuff tears in athletes. Orthop Clin North Am 4:721, 1973

Bernhang AM, Dehner W, Fogerty C: Tennis elbow: a biomechanical approach. J Sports Med 2:235, 1974

Blair W, Hanley S: Stress fracture of the proximal fibula. Am J Sports Med. 8:212, 1980

Brodelius A: Osteoarthrosis of the talar joints in footballers and ballet dancers. Acta Orthop Scand 30:309, 1961

Buckwalter JA: Articular cartilage. p. 349. In Evarts CM (ed): Instructional Course Lectures AAOS. CV Mosby, St. Louis, 1983

Christiansen T, Wilson K: Facial injuries in sports. Minn Med 66:29, 1983

Corringan B: Musculo-skeletal complications of jogging. Br J Sports Med 14:37, 1980

Currey JD. Changes in the impact energy absorption of bone with age. J Biomech 12:459, 1979

Davies JE: The spine in sport—injuries, prevention and treatment. Br J Sports Med 14:18, 1980

Davies JE. Sports injuries and society. Br J Sports Med 15:80, 1981.

DeHaven KE, Evarts CM: Throwing injuries of the elbow in athletes. Orthop Clin North Am 4:801, 1973

Dias LS, Tachdjian MO: Physical injuries of the ankle in children. Clin Orthop 136:230, 1978

Drez D, Jr., Young JC, Johnston RD, Parker WD: Metatarsal stress fractures. Am J Sports Med 8:123, 1980

Dugan RC, D'ambrosia R: Fibular stress fractures in runners. J Fam Pract 17:415, 1983

Eggold JF: Orthotics in the prevention of runner's overuse injuries. Phys Sports Med 9:125, 1981

Frankel VH, Hang YS: Recent advances in the biomechanics of sports injuries. Acta Orthop Scand 46:484, 1975

Frost HM: An Introduction to Biomechanics. Charles C. Thomas, Springfield, Ill., 1973

Gainor BJ, Piotrowski G, Puhl J et al: The throw: biomechanics and acute injury. Am J Sports Med 8:114, 1980

Garrick JG: Ankle injuries: frequency and mechanism of injury. Athletic Training 10:109, 1975

Garrick JG: Sports medicine. Pediatr Clin North Am 24:737, 1977

Garrick JG: An introduction to orthopedics. p. 187. In Strauss RH (ed): Sports Medicine and Physiology. WB Saunders, Philadelphia, 1979

Gerberich SG, Priest JD, Grafft J, Siebert RC: Injuries to the brain and spinal cord; assessment, emergency care, and prevention. Minn Med 65:691, 1982

Greenwald AS: Ankle joint mechanics. p. 253. In Yablon IG, Segal D, Leach RE (eds): Ankle Injuries. Churchill Livingstone, New York, 1983

Gregersen HN: Fractures of the humerus from muscular violence. Acta Orthop Scand 42:506, 1971

Gurdijian ES, Lissner HR, Patrick LM. Protection of the head and neck in sports. JAMA 182:509, 1982

Harrington IJ. Biomechanics of joint injuries. p. 31. Gozna ER (ed): Biomechanics of Musculoskeletal Injury. Williams and Wilkins, Baltimore, 1982

Harvey JS, Jr.: Overuse syndromes in young athletes. Pediatr Clin North Am 29:1369, 1982

Henderson J. The athletes dilemma. J Am Podiatry Assoc, 64:124, 1974

Hirsch C: Biomechanics in motor skeletal trauma J Trauma 10:997, 1970

Hogue CC: Injury in latelife. II: prevention. J Am Geriatr Soc 30:276, 1982

Hunter LY, Andrews JR, Claney WG et al: Common orthopedic problems of female athletes. p. 126. In Frankel VH (ed): Instructional Course Lectures AAOS. CV Mosby, St. Louis, 1982

Jobe FW, Jobe CM: Painful athletic injuries of the shoulder. Clin Orthop 173:117, 1983

Kennedy JC, Hawkins RJ: Swimmer's shoulder. Phys Sports Med 2:35, 1974

Kleiger B: Mechanisms of ankle injury. Orthop Clin North Am 5:127, 1974

Krissoff WB, Ferris WD: Runner's injuries. Phys Sports Med 7:55, 1979

Kuprian W: Physical Therapy for Sports. WB Saunders, Philadelphia, 1982

Larson RL, McMahon RO: The epiphyses and the childhood athlete. JAMA 196:607, 1966

Liljedahl SO: Common injuries in connection with conditioning exercise. Scand J Rehab Med 3:1, 1971

Lipscomb AB: Baseball pitching injuries in growing athletes. J Sports Med 3:25, 1975

Markham DE: Sports injuries: causes. Br J Hosp Med 29:209, 1983

McLatchie GR, Miller JH, Morris EW: Combined force injury of the elbow joint—the mechanism clarified Br J Sports Med 13:176, 1979

Medhat MA, Redford JB: Knee injuries: Damage from running and related sports. J Kans Med Soc 84:379, 1983

Micheli LJ: Overuse injuries in children's sports: the overuse factor. Orthop Clin North Am 14:337, 1983

Mucha P, Jr.: Abdominal injuries. Minn Med 66:93, 1983

Nicholas JA: Athletics injuries to the upper extremity of adolescents. p. 101. In Symposium on Sports Medicine AAOS. CV Mosby, St. Louis, 1969

Nicholas JA: Ankle injuries in athletes. Orthop Clin North Am 5:153, 1974

Noble CA: Iliotibial band friction syndrome in runners. Am J Sports Med 8:232, 1980

Orva S, Puranen J: Exertion injuries in adolescent athletes. Br J Sports Med 12:4, 1978

Orava S, Saarela J: Exertion injuries to young athletes. Am J Sports Med 6:68, 1978

Orava S: Stress fractures. Br J Sports Med 14:40, 1980

Pavlov H, Nelson TL, Warren RF et al: Stress fractures of the pubic ramus. J Bone Joint Surg 64A:1020, 1982

Priest JD: Elbow injuries in sports. Minn Med 65:543–545, 1982

Quigley TB: Common musculoskeletal problems. p. 179. In Strauss RH (ed): Sports Medicine and Physiology. WB Saunders, Philadelphia, 1979

Quigley TB: Injuries to soft tissues. p. 179. In Strauss RH (ed): Sports Medicine and Physiology. WB Saunders, Philadelphia, 1979

Radin EL, Paul IL, Rose RM: Role of mechanical factors in pathogenesis of primary osteoarthritis. Lancet 1:519, 1972

Rodgers MM, Cavanaugh PR: Glossary of biomechanical terms, concepts, and units. Phys Ther 64:1886, 1984

Roy S, Irvin R: Sports Medicine: Prevention, Evaluation, Management, and Rehabilitation. Prentice Hall, Englewood Cliffs, 1983

Siffert RS, Levy RN: Athletic injuries in children. Pediatr Clin North Am 12:1027, 1965

Smillie IS: Diseases of the Knee Joint. 2nd Ed. Churchill Livingtone, New York 1980

Subotnik SI: A biomechanical approach to running injuries. Ann NY Acad Sci 301:888, 1977

Subotnik SI: Podiatric aspects of children in sports. J Am Podiatry Assoc 69:443, 1979

Teitz CC: Sports medicine concerts in dance and gymnastics. Pediatr Clin North Am 29:1399, 1982

Temple C: Sports injuries: hazards of jogging and marathon running. Br J Hosp Med 29:237, 1983

Vidt L, Marks J, Brown F: Fatigue fractures: a literature review. J Am Podiatry Assoc 68:326, 1978

Voloshin A, Wosk J. Influence of artificial shock absorbers on human gait Clin Orthop 160:52, 1981

Walter NE, Wolf MD: Stress fractures in young athletes. Am J Sports Med 5:165, 1977

White AA, III, Panjabe MM: Clinical Biomechanics of the Spine. JB Lippincott, Philadelphia, 1978

Wilkins KE: The uniqueness of the athlete: musculoskeletal injuries. Am J Sports Med 8:377, 1980

Williams JGP: Wear and tear injuries in athletes—an overview. Br J Sports Med 12:211, 1979

Williams JGP: Biomechanical factors in spinal injuries. Br J Sports Med 14:14, 1980

Worthen BM, Yanklowitz BAD: The pathophysiology and treatment of stress fracture in military personnel. J Am Podiatry Assoc 68:317, 1978

7 | Triage

Donna B. Bernhardt

The past decade has been punctuated by an emerging public consciousness concerning health and wellness that has spawned an increasing interest in the benefits of physical fitness. The result has been an expansion of available athletic activities and a growing number of participants in lifetime sports pursuits. Despite the sophistication of medical care, athletic equipment, and rules of play, the volume of activities and participants and the intensity of modern training techniques have led to an overall increase in athletic injuries.

An athletic injury, a disruption of tissue continuity that causes a restriction or cessation of normal activity or sports participation, results from the application of forces in excess of the body's adaptive capacities. Although prevention is the ideal method of injury management, prompt and accurate triage care is essential for an effective system of medical service.

The word "triage" has a French derivation that means sorting and choice selection. The modernized definition connotes an integral process in which emergency patients are introduced into a health care system. The personnel performing triage become the stimulus for initiation of a care flow pattern that includes early recognition and definition of the problem, determination of the urgency of care, development and prioritization of treatment plans, initiation of the most appropriate course of action, and documentation of the entire process.

Triage is only one important step in the process of total maintenance of the athletic participant that includes rehabilitation (reconditioning), organization and administration of services, and education of the athlete and all related personnel.

ASSESSMENT PROCESS

Accurate initial assessment of a sports-related injury, which is vital to medical care, establishes the type and severity of the injury and the course of subsequent care. Further injury or delayed recovery can result from inadequate or inaccurate immediate evaluation.

Initial assessment is best made at the moment of injury, when the athlete experiences the least discomfort and before signs and symptoms are masked by pain, edema, inflammatory response, and protection muscle spasm. The ideal location for initial assessment is the site of the injury. A cursory on-location assessment of the nature and severity of the injury provides a more accurate basis for decisionmaking.

Accurate assessment requires a thorough knowledge of anatomy and physiology because each potentially involved structure or system must be isolated and evaluated. An organized, systematic evaluation sequence reduces potential for errors in judgment. Providers of triage must be adept and honest assessing their evaluative skills. They must keep current on injury assessment skills and be familiar with medical symptoms (subjective evidence) and signs (objective evidence). A comprehensive knowledge of additional diagnostic procedures is not vital, but triage providers should be familiar with current procedures and their availability to make appropriate facility referrals.

A knowledge of the athlete, including personality, current medical status, and pertinent past medical history, enhances assessment. Understanding the basic biomechanical fundamentals and the physiological and psychological demands of a sport is an asset when determining the mechanism of injury or the appropriateness of returning the activity.

Triage is most effective if the provider is calm and patient. Calmness conveys competence and control of the situation and serves to defuse anxiety of the team, spectators, and victim. Patience produces a more accurate and complete evaluation. Experience, gained only through practice, breeds confidence, efficiency, and accuracy, but only if the practitioner is open to continual learning. As long as there is ongoing education, experience has no substitute.

ASSESSMENT PROCEDURES

In addition to triage personnel at athletic events, a physician should be present to provide higher levels of medical intervention. Access to a telephone provides immediate linkage to emergency vehicles and care facilities. An emergency vehicle on the scene facilitates speed of medical attention. The availability of specialized equipment and supplies on the sideline or in a nearby facility is imperative to both adequate evaluation and immediate first aid. A list of suggested materials is outlined in Table 7-1.

The evaluation is performed to determine the type, location, and severity of the injury. Injuries are classified either by priority of care or solution indicated. Table 7-2 outlines both classification systems and their interaction.

In assessing the injury, the provider must blend subjective information from the injured party or an observer with objective data from the actual examination to derive the probable cause and result. Experience and reevaluation substantiate the initial assessment. Thorough assessment consists of two parts: the primary basic assessment and the secondary systems survey.

Table 7-1. Suggested Triage Equipment

Triage Kit		Equipment
Acetaminophen tablets	Forceps	Cervical and spinal boards
Adhesive tape ($\frac{1}{2}$-inch and $1\frac{1}{2}$-	Fungicide	Crutches
inch)	Germicide	Ice chest
Alcohol	Heel cups	Splints (air or prefabricated)
Ammonia	Ice bags	
Analgesic balm	Medicated ointment	
Ankle wraps	Mirror	
Antacid tablets	Moleskin	
Antiglare salve	Nail clippers	
Antiseptic soap	Oral screw	
Aspirin	Pen	
Baking soda	Pins	
Adhesive strips (including	Prewrap	
butterflies and steri-strips)	Razor	
Calamine lotion	Reflex hammer	
Callous file	Salt tablets	
Cotton and cotton-tipped	Scalpel	
applicators	Scissors (regular, bandage,	
Drinking cups	surgical)	
Elastic bandages and tape	Sterile gauze and pads	
Epinephrine syringe	Tape adherent and remover	
(precalibrated)	Thermometer	
Eye dropper and eye cup	Tongue depressors	
Felt and foam	Triangular bandage or slings	
Flashlight	Petroleum jelly	
Flexible collodion		

Table 7-2. Injury Classification System

Priority of Care	Solution
First	
Immediate threat to life	Physician and hospital referral
Medical intervention essential within	
minutes or a few hours	
Second	
Threat to life and well-being present but not	Physican and hospital referral or sideline and
immediate	training room evaluation
Medical intervention urgent within several	
hours	
Third	
No threat to life	Sideline and training room evaluation or
Medical intervention necessary but not	return to play
urgent	

Primary Assessment

Primary basic assessment is the evaluation of the basic life-support mechanisms: airway, breathing, and circulation. Inadequacy of any of these conditions is potentially life-threatening and requires immediate and effective intervention. The primary assessment is completed easily and quickly, often before reaching the athlete. If the injured athlete is talking and conscious, it can be that he or she has adequate aeration and circulation. If the athlete is unconscious, a total primary assessment must be made at the site.

The environment and any immediate dangers, such as electric wiring, should be observed while going to the site. Level of consciousness, body position, and hemorrhage should be noted immediately upon reaching the injured person. Clothing and face guards may need to be cut away. Helmets should not be removed if there is any suspicion of head or spinal injury.

The airway can be obstructed by anything that blocks the passage of air through the trachea into the lungs. Foreign objects, such as dental appliances, chewing gum, and mouth guards, can block the airway, but the most common obstruction is the tongue, especially in the unconscious victim. The tongue falls toward the back of the throat and blocks the glottis. Because the tongue is attached to the mandible, forward motion of this bone usually lifts the tongue away from the posterior pharynx. Any one of three methods—head tilt with neck lift, head tilt with chin lift, or jaw thrust—will create forward motion of the lower jaw if there is sufficient tone in the jaw musculature. The choice of method depends on the injury. The jaw thrust maneuver should be used whenever a cervical spine trauma is suspected. When the airway has been positioned by head tilt or jaw thrust, the triage provider should observe for chest motion. If air exchange is noted, breathing should be monitored; if not, the jaw or head should be repositioned. If no exchange occurs following repositioning, the provider should attempt to force four quick breaths into the victim's mouth. Lack of air exchange now indicates an occluded airway that must be cleared immediately. The mouth should be cleared if an object is apparent. Otherwise, the American Heart Association method of back blows and abdominal or chest thrusts should be used, with repeated attempts at aeration until the airway is cleared. Once the airway is cleared, spontaneous breathing should be monitored closely. If apnea persists, as in cases of cardiac arrest, intrathoracic injury, or anaphylaxis, appropriate techniques of artificial ventilation should be instituted.

Cardiac function and resultant systemic circulation are evaluated by assessing a pulse. In most emergency situations, a central pulse, the carotid, is evaluated for presence, quality, and rhythm. If no pulse is noted, appropriate emergency techniques of artificial circulation should be initiated by one or two rescuers. If there is a pulse, circulatory status should be monitored closely.

If breathing and circulation are absent, cardiopulmonary resuscitation procedures must be instituted immediately and continued until cardiorespiratory efforts are spontaneous or until transport is completed and hospital care is initiated.

The primary survey is summarized in Figure 7-1. When the primary assessment is complete and all basic life-support systems are normalized, the secondary survey should begin.

Secondary Survey

The secondary survey consists of a concise but thorough evaluation to define the nature, location, and degree of all injuries. This assessment can be made at the injury site, on the sidelines, or both. The significant components

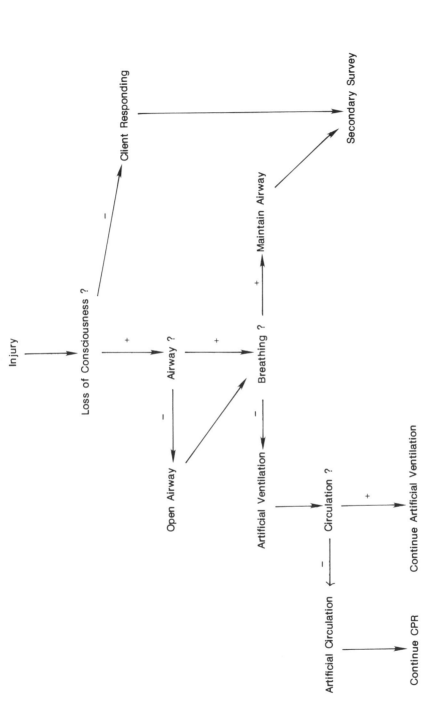

Fig. 7-1. Steps in primary basic assessment.

of the secondary survey are a history, observation, palpation, and neurological screening and special stress testing. Which components to include and where the survey is conducted depend on the nature and degree of the injury.

The history, the subjective part of the secondary survey, should include as much information as possible about the injury and its occurrence. The information can be compiled by questioning the injured person or witnesses. Because the history provides important clues as to which structures might be involved and hence which objective evaluative tools may be indicated, posing well-phrased and pointed questions is vital. Questions should be simple, concise, and direct and asked one at a time, in a logical fashion. Specifically, the following should be defined: chief complaint; behavior of the symptom; location and radiation of the symptom; mode of onset (gradual versus sudden); severity (on a scale of 1 to 10); date of onset, frequency, and time of occurrence; mechanism of injury (if known); functional alterations; related symptoms; and past injuries to the area. A decision regarding probable injury and appropriate or immediate treatment strategies should be made only after all questions have been answered.

Observation of the injury process, the scene of the injury, and associated apparatus or equipment may give clues to the nature of the injury. The athlete's level of consciousness and response to the injury should be noted, as should body or segment position and posture, body motion, obvious hemorrhage, deformity, swelling, or discoloration, and signs of trauma, such as abrasions. The area should be examined and compared with the noninvolved side, if possible.

The injured area should be palpated gently. Palpation should begin on a distant site so the athlete's confidence is secured and the involved areas become relaxed. Palpation can define the location of pain, degree and type of swelling, temperature and texture of an area, presence of muscle spasm, tissue continuity and deformity, neurovascular level of function, and abnormal motion or sensation.

Neurological screening and special stress testing provide insight into tissue integrity and further delineate the area and severity of insult. These tests should not be used where fracture or dislocation is suspected.

In neurological screening, active, functional, and resistive motions are utilized to evaluate the integrity and innervation of contractile tissues, such as muscles and tendons. Pain during any of these motions implicates the contractile elements as the problem source. Active and functional motions, which produce the least stress because the athlete can control the velocity and excursion of the movement, can be used to document pain-free range of motion, with the intensity of functional activities increased until the extent of injury is ascertained. Resistive motion, applied either isometrically or throughout a range of available motion, can be used to define muscle strength and extent of injury. Sport-specific function should be assessed and normalized before the athlete returns to activity.

Specific stress testing consists of passive, arthrokinematic (joint-play) movement and stress application designed to assess the integrity of noncontractile tissues, such as ligament, joint capsule, bone, and bursa. This testing

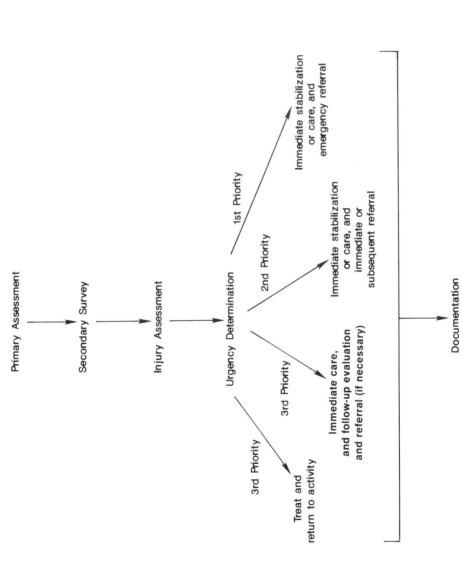

Fig. 7-2. Assessment tree.

Table 7-3. Priority Determination

First Priority	Second Priority	Third Priority
Cardiac or respiratory arrest	Loss of consciousness	Other musculoskeletal
Massive hemorrhage	Myocardial infarction	injuries
Shock	Facial or EENT injury	Abrasions
Anaphylaxis	Head injury	Blisters
Heat stroke	Seizures	Lacerations
Choking	Bleeding	
Hypothermia	Burns	
	Spinal insult	
	Visceral injury	
	Asthma	
	Fractures or dislocations	
	Thermal stress	
	Diabetic hyperglycemia or	
	hypoglycemia	

reveals instability, laxity, and pain. These passive motions frequently reproduce the mechanism of injury and permit evaluation of available pain-free os-
teokinematic range of motion. Occurrence of pain implicates either noncontractile tissue or joint surfaces.

Interpretation and Intervention

When the primary assessment and secondary survey have been completed,
problems should be listed and an assessment of the injury made. Based on the
assessment, intervention should be prioritized and implemented. Figure 7-2
outlines the assessment sequence.

Documentation

Documentation facilitates referral and management and protects against
liability. Complete records are an outstanding teaching tool and can provide
data for retrospective analysis of injury patterns and intervention effectiveness
and other research.

Documentation of the assessment should be clear, concise, and legible and
should summarize all important data. A standard injury report form makes
documentation fast, accurate, and thorough.

ASSESSMENT AND INTERVENTION STRATEGIES IN
SPECIFIC ATHLETIC INJURIES

First Priority

Cardiopulmonary Arrest.   The cardiac and respiratory systems are evaluated in the primary assessment.

Respiratory arrest most frequently results from airway obstruction, but head trauma, cervical injury, maxillofacial or thoracic trauma, cerebral vascular accident, or myocardial infarction can cause arrest. Cardiac arrest can occur secondary to respiratory failure, ventricular fibrillation, or thoracic trauma. Regardless of the cause, the injured person should be supine for evaluation and treatment. If the person is in any other position, the triage provider should log-roll him or her, stabilizing the head and cervical regions and other severely injured areas. The level of consciousness should be established and coloration of lips, tongue, or nail beds noted—cyanosis indicates inadequate or absent aeration. The pattern, symmetry, and sound of respiration should be noted—these may indicate the degree and cause of airway obstruction.

Interventions should be artificial ventilation and/or circulation, as recommended by the American Heart Association. In the case of a flail chest secondary to multiple rib fractures, a wide bandage can be applied transthoracically, or manual or sandbag stabilization instituted, to stabilize the thorax. If a bandage is used, it should be applied loosely to prevent rib pressure with subsequent lung puncture. If the pneumothorax is open (communicating), the wound should be covered with a sterile material.

Emergency resuscitation should continue until the physiological systems respond or until the person is pronounced dead by a physician. Efforts should be maintained during transfer.

Choking.   Choking can result from partial or complete airway obstruction or aspiration of food, liquid, or objects. The tongue can occlude the airway in an unconscious person. Signs of choking include violent coughing, labored and noisy respiration, cyanosis, and eventual apnea and loss of consciousness. In the case of apnea or unconsciousness, the airway should be cleared as outlined in the section on primary assessment. If the athlete is conscious and has good air exchange (can still speak or cough to some audible degree), he or she should not be interfered with unless apnea or loss of consciousness occurs. If the person is conscious with no air exchange (cyanotic, no cough, grasps throat), back blows and abdominal or chest thrusts should be used until the airway clears.

Anaphylaxis.   Anaphylaxis is an immediate allergic response leading to local or systemic reactions. Local responses include itching, uticaria, and angioedema. Systemic responses are faintness, dypsnea, bronchospasm, and respiratory collapse. The most effective treatment is prevention by desensitization or allergen control. In the event of a large localized or a systemic reaction, immediate referral is indicated. Precalibrated syringes of epinephrine can be injected intramuscularly if the individual or triage provider has the medication and the proper instruction.

Hemorrhage.   Both internal and external hemorrhage can result from trauma. Signs of internal hemorrhage include cold, clammy skin, rapid pulse and respiration, palpable pain and tenderness, restlessness, excessive thirst, blood in the urine or stool.

When internal hemorrhage is suspected, emergency medical care is indicated. The victim should be transported in a supine and well-supported position.

No fluids should be given, and the victim should be observed for shock or arrest.

External hemorrhage must be stopped immediately, before emergency referral, preferably with direct pressure over the site with a sterile cloth. The area should be elevated. Additional layers should be applied when the first layer is soaked; removing the first layer could dislodge clots. If bleeding does not stop, arterial pressure point compression may be required. A tourniquet should be applied and time of application noted only for severe, uncontrollable, life-threatening hemorrhage.

If the hemorrhage is caused by a protruding foreign object, the object should be left in place and stabilized before transport. Once hemorrhage is controlled, the wound should be covered to prevent further contamination. The area should be immobilized, especially if a fracture exists. The victim should be monitored continuously for shock or arrest.

Shock.   Any significant injury can result in shock, or cardiovascular collapse or depression. Important signs include: rapid, weak pulse and respiration; cold, clammy skin; profuse sweating; nausea; dull, dilated pupils; low blood pressure, altered sensorium. Shock can be life-threatening but can be reversed by immediate intervention.

The individual should be lying down, preferably with the lower extremities elevated if injury is not aggravated. Obvious bleeding should be stopped. Body temperature should be maintained to prevent chilling, but active warming shunts blood to the periphery and is contraindicated. Oral fluids should not be administered unless medical attention is delayed. Immediate medical assistance or transport is vital.

Heatstroke.   Heatstroke, failure of the thermoregulatory system, causes death if not treated immediately. Signs characteristically include elevated temperature (>105°F); red, hot, dry skin; strong and rapid pulse; lack of sweating. The body temperature must be reduced as quickly as possible. A heatstroke victim should be moved from sunlight and any clothing and equipment removed. The body should be cooled by cold water immersion, ice or cold packing, or cold water or alcohol sponging. Emergency assistance should be sought.

Hypothermia.   Hypothermia is thermoregulatory failure when core temperature falls below 95°F. Early signs include shivering, depressed respiration, and slow and erratic pulse. As hypothermia progresses, the mental state alters and confusion and incoordination develop. Finally, rigidity, coma, and collapse results. A person with hypothermia should be taken to a warm area and stripped of wet or frozen clothing. Blankets should be used to warm the victim and emergency assistance should be sought.

Second Priority

Loss of Consciousness.   Loss of consciousness is defined as an inability to respond to any sensory stimuli, except pain. Causes of unconsciousness can be head injury, heatstroke, hypothermia, diabetes, epilepsy, or cerebral or cardiac malfunction.

If an athlete appears unresponsive, loud or repeated verbal stimuli should be used to evaluate the level of consciousness and the person should be shaken gently. If no response is elicited, primary basic assessment should be initiated, always assuming the possibility of a head or neck injury.

Once the basic systems are stabilized, a history should be taken from observers. Level of consciousness should be determined by length and depth of unconscious state. Abnormal position or posture of head, neck, and extremities; hemorrhage; and rate, character, and pattern of respiratory efforts should be observed. The pupils should be examined for size, equality, and response to light. Abnormality of posture, respiration, or pupils is a sign of serious damage and warrants immediate referral.

Skin color is an indicator of adequate blood flow and blood oxygenation. The face, neck, upper chest, and lips or tongue should be examined for rubor, pallor, or cyanosis. Rubor indicates heatstroke or high blood pressure. Pallor indicates hemorrhage or shock. Cyanosis indicates heart failure or respiratory inadequacy.

Signs of trauma to the ears or nose such as lacerations, deformity, discoloration, ecchymosis, or discharge suggest a skull fracture.

Presence, quality, and rate of pulse, blood pressure, and temperature should be assessed. Low pulse or blood pressure suggests lack of blood volume or circulating sufficiency. Increasing pressure with low pulse rate indicates cerebral hemorrhage.

The scalp, neck, and hairline should be palpated gently for deformities, depressions, or blood. Reactivity to pain can be evaluated by pin prick, sternal compression, or nipple or calf pressure. A lack of response may indicate coma or spinal cord injury. Postural response suggests brain damage. Motion and stress tests are contraindicated.

A person who regains consciousness in less than 1 minute with no cardiovascular compromise should be monitored for potential head injury. Extended unconsciousness necessitates emergency transport and care.

Seizures.   Head trauma, epilepsy, and metabolic abnormality can cause seizure. Most seizures are self-limited but may be characterized by uncontrollable motion, irregular respiration, loss of bowel and bladder control, and teeth clenching. Management is primarily protective. The area should be cleared to protect the person's body. If the mouth is open, a soft bite stick should be inserted between the teeth; the mouth should not be forced open. Following seizure, airway and breathing should be checked. The person should remain lying, preferably on one side to prevent aspiration. The person should be referred for subsequent evaluation.

Head Injury.   Head injury includes damage to the skull, scalp, or brain secondary to application of sudden force to the head. Scalp lacerations or contusions, skull fractures, cerebral concussion, contusion, and hemorrhage may result.

The primary basic life support systems must be evaluated and stabilized. The secondary survey must establish a neurological base line upon which to monitor physical signs and symptoms over a period of time. Improvement from the base line suggests no additional intracranial involvement; deterioration suggests increased involvement and mandates referral for medical treatment.

A history should be taken to the assess mechanism of injury, occurrence of seizure or loss of consciousness, and any changing clinical signs. Level of consciousness should be assessed by monitoring orientation, alertness, responsiveness, and awareness of persons, time, and place. Presence of amnesia suggests concussion or contusion. Altered consciousness indicates cerebral damage. Other symptoms of intracranial injury are headache, pain, sensory changes, tinnitus, nausea or vomiting, and double or blurred vision.

The victim should be observed for speech difficulties, attempted or abnormal bodily movement, weakness or paralysis, and change in level of consciousness. Pupil size, reactivity, and symmetry should be evaluated and gaze and eye motion assessed for smoothness, coordination, symmetry, and control. Respiratory function, signs of trauma, and pulse should be assessed as in an unconscious person. Coordination should be serially monitored with a test such as the Romberg test. Sensorimotor function and the quality of motion and gait should be assessed. Ataxia, tone changes, tremor or motion disturbance are suggestive of cerebellar damage.

If the athlete continues to improve, he or she should be monitored until all signs and symptoms are normalized. On release, a list of signs suggesting intracranial damage should be given to the athlete or the athlete's family or a friend with instructions to contact a physician if any occur. If the athlete does not improve or deteriorates, he or she should be referred for medical treatment.

Spinal Insult. Spinal injuries can occur to any area of the spinal column as a result of forced or abnormal motion, a sudden fall, or an outside blow. These injuries can be the most serious, so on-site evaluation should err on the conservative side to prevent any further damage.

The primary survey should be completed, especially if cervical lesions are suspected. If the athlete is unconscious, he or she should be managed as if there is a spinal cord injury. If the airway must be cleared, a jaw–thrust maneuver should be used. The athlete should be moved only if absolutely necessary, and then with extreme care: the body should be rolled as a unit with the entire spine protected, especially the suspect area. Any transfer should be on a spine board with the head and neck careful stabilized manually or with sandbags or a cervical collar. Immediate medical attention is indicated.

After the primary assessment, if the athlete is conscious, the secondary survey can be initiated, but the athlete still should be handled as if there is a spinal injury. Initially, the evaluation should be conducted with the athlete in his or her original injured position. The airway, breathing, and circulation should be monitored continuously.

A history should be taken to find the mechanism of injury and the forces applied and whether the injury is a result of an acute trauma or repetitive chronic stress—sprains, strains, and fractures result from sudden trauma, and spondylolysis usually develops secondary to repetitive insult. A report of previous injury or symptoms will clarify this. The athlete should be asked whether he or she feels pain or felt unusual sensations, such as burning, a sharp stab of pain, or tingling and numbness, during or after the insult.

Signs of trauma, obvious spinal deformity, and the position of the head, trunk, and extremities should be noted. If the athlete is moving, the quality and location of motion should be assessed, with particular attention to any area that is immobile.

Palpation is extremely important in assessing spinal cord injury. A loss or decrease in sensorimotor function is the most reliable indicator of cord damage; this should be evaluated thoroughly and both sides compared. Motor function is evaluated most safely with active motion of small distal joints and isometric contraction of larger, more proximal joints. This method permits accurate assessment with no risk of further damage through body movement. Sensation of light touch and noxious stimuli (pin prick) on the extremities should be assessed with an attempt to clarify dermatomal or peripheral nerve patterns of sensory alteration. Any paraesthesies should be localized and noted. Any alteration in sensorimotor function indicates cord or peripheral nerve damage and requires immediate medical attention.

If the sensorimotor system is intact, the athlete still may have serious bone damage. Transport and further sideline assessment will depend on the situation. If a serious injury is suspected, more thorough medical evaluation should be obtained if any suspicion of serious injury exists. Once it is clear that the injury is not potentially serious or unstable, posture, pain and tenderness, neuromotor function, gait, and functional activities should be evaluated more thoroughly. The athlete should return to the sport only if results of all assessments are good and all signs and symptoms resolve in a short period.

Visceral Injury.   Most athletic injuries to the thorax and abdomen are superficial, but there is a possibility of serious internal injury, especially in contact sports. The most frequent cause of injury is a direct blow to the area. Because the internal organs are essential for respiration and circulation, any blow resulting in serious injury can be life-threatening. Internal injuries can become serious very quickly, so immediate assessment and management are vital. Follow-up evaluation is necessary in any case of a severe blow, even if no initial signs exist, to detect slowly developing problems. No food, liquid, or medication should be ingested in any intrathoracic or intraabdominal injury because medication may mask pain or symptoms and food may aggravate symptoms or complicate any necessary surgical procedure.

Once the primary assessment has been made, a history should be taken to elucidate the mechanism of injury and precise location of contact. Behavior and location of pain are very important, because visceral pain is often poorly localized and referred distally (i.e., bladder–upper thigh, liver–right shoulder, spleen–left shoulder and upper arm, and intestines and back). Additional symptoms, such as crepitation on respiration, abdominal muscle spasm or rigidity, nausea and vomiting, or difficulty in breathing, should be noted.

The position and movement of the athlete may indicate what area is being protected. Depth, pattern, symmetry, and rate of respiration should be assessed to evaluate for rib injury or lung damage. Tracheal deviation from the midline, which may indicate thoracic damage, should be noted. Obvious signs of trauma should be evaluated. The vital signs should be monitored continuously, because cardiorespiratory arrest or shock may develop secondary to any internal injury.

The person should be palpated gently to confirm any findings. The thorax should be palpated to assess symmetry of respiration and obvious deformity, crepitus, or swelling. The abdomen should be palpated with the lower extremities in a flexed position for relaxation and abdominal tenderness, rigidity, guarding, or deformity and rebound tenderness noted.

If internal injury is indicated, the athlete should be referred immediately for medical evaluation and care. Persons with a thoracic injury should be transported in a semi-reclining position to ease respiration; with a suspected rib fracture in such a way as to avoid puncturing the lung; and with abdominal injuries in a supine position with the hips and knees flexed. Increasing respiratory distress or tracheal shift may indicate a pneumothorax and should be treated as an emergency.

Delayed symptoms frequently develop hours, days, or weeks after initial insult; thus any unusual signs or symptoms should be reported immediately.

Genital injury is uncommon, especially in female athletes. In male athletes, direct blow to the genitalia may result in severe muscular spasm. Two methods may relieve this spasm: the knees may be flexed to the chest, or the sitting athlete may be lifted under the axilla (2 to 3 inches from ground) and then dropped. If symptoms persist, further medical attention is indicated.

Facial, Eye, Ear, and Nose Injury. Injuries to the face, eyes, ears, nose, and throat are common although protective devices have reduced the frequency and severity of these injuries. An injury in these areas could indicate head or neck injury. Careful evaluation and management especially important for good cosmetic results.

When primary basic systems are cleared and stabilized, the secondary survey can begin. A history should be taken to define the injuries, force, and resulting symptoms. The victim should be observed for signs of trauma, unusual bleeding, deformity, and presense of foreign bodies and palpated to localize the symptoms and reveal crepitation, deformity, increased mobility, or swelling.

Jaw or cheek. Asymmetry, point tenderness, pain on motion, and malocclusion are indicators of fracture and necessitate medical attention. Ice and a jaw sling can be used to reduce pain and edema and stabilize the area.

Nose. Nosebleed, deformity, tenderness, pain with motion, and abnormal mobility are indicators of nasal fracture and necessitate medical attention. Nosebleeds should be controlled immediately, usually with a nasal pinch and ice. Packing may be necessary if bleeding will not stop after 20 minutes. The person should be transported in a sitting position so the blood is not aspirated.

Ear. External and internal structures of the ear should be examined with an otoscope and good illumination. Hemorrhage or cerebrospinal otorrhea indicate skull fracture, which demands immediate referral. Defective hearing, vertigo, and nausea are symptoms of middle or inner ear defects and require medical attention. Injuries to external structures can be managed with ice, compression, and protective padding. Referral may be indicated for medication or decompression therapy.

Teeth. Damaged teeth should be checked by a dentist. Immediate referral is necessary for severe pain or for a tooth that is knocked out. When a tooth is knocked out, it should be cleaned and reimplanted immediately or saved in a moist cloth during transport to a dentist, which should occur within $\frac{1}{2}$ hour. If a tooth is chipped or cracked, referral is indicated but is not urgent. A loosened tooth should be protected from forceful biting during play.

Eye. Eye injuries should be screened for possible referral immediately, before swelling occurs. The account of injury and chief complaint define the potential problem. The eye should be observed for deformity, hemorrhage, and trauma. Visual acuity, pupil size and reactivity, and eye motion should be assessed. The eyelid should be examined gently with a cotton-tipped applicator for the presence of a foreign body. Foreign bodies usually can be removed by tearing or irrigation. If it cannot be removed or if irritation persists after removal, referral is indicated. Small lacerations of soft tissue near the eye should be cleaned and approximated. Large soft tissue lacerations or lacerations of the eyeball should be referred. One or both eyes should be patched before transfer to minimize eye motion and stress.

If the person wears contact lenses, they may be displaced on the eye or, in the case of injury, may need to be removed. Drops should not be used in penetrating injuries.

Myocardial Infarction. Heart attacks during sports activities are uncommon. Although no symptoms occur in some cases, dyspnea, angina, left shoulder and arm pain, neck and jaw pain, and chest tightness indicate ischemia and infarction. A history of cardiac problems coupled with decreased heart sounds and lowered blood pressure is suggestive of myocardial problems. Individuals with these signs should have immediate and continuous cardiorespiratory assessment and stabilization while being transported for further medical evaluation.

Asthma. Participants in sports may have either asthma or exercise-induced asthma. Asthmatic exacerbation should be prevented with medication, breathing control, and use of a face mask to warm air. Persons with asthmatic difficulties may exhibit dyspnea, wheezing, or abnormal breath sounds. Relaxation and breathing exercises may improve respiratory control. Ingestion or inhalation of prescribed medications and adequate hydration are indicated. If the exacerbation is moderate to severe, referral to a physician may be necessary.

Diabetes. A person with well-controlled diabetes usually can participate in athletic activities without difficulty, but if insulin levels become too low (hyperglycemia) or too high (hypoglycemia), diabetic coma or shock, respectively, can occur.

Symptoms of diabetic coma are stomach ache, lethargy, confusion, elevated pulse, fruity breath secondary to ketosis, and eventual coma. The immediate treatment of choice is administration of insulin by injection or immediate referral.

Diabetic shock is characterized by fatigue, irritability, slurred speech, headache, hunger, lack of coordination, and normal pulse and breathing. Eventual unconsciousness can follow. Insulin overdose, too much exercise, or too little food can cause diabetic shock; it is more common than diabetic coma. Immediate treatment is glucose ingestion in the form of fruit juice, glucose solution, or food high in sugar (candy). The person should be referred for adjustment of insulin dosage.

Burns.   Severe burns, rare in athletics, can result from lightning. It is imperative to stabilize the basic life systems. Jewelry, clothing, and equipment should be removed before swelling occurs. The victim should be lain flat and covered and kept warm. Dry, clean dressings should be applied to affected areas before transport. Fluids in small amounts should be dispensed to conscious patients to maintain hydration.

Thermal Stress Syndromes.   The heat syndromes resulting from thermal exposure include heat exhaustion and heat cramps. Both result from strenuous activity in hot and humid weather with secondary loss of body fluid and a thermoregulatory derangement.

Heat cramps are painful spasms of skeletal muscles secondary to a fluid volume problem. They accompany strenuous activity and profuse perspiration. Immediate symptoms include muscle cramping and pain with functional limitation. Other physiological systems are usually normal. The management of choice is rehydration by liberal ingestion of fluids (primarily water) and reduction of spasm by slow stretching or firm pressure.

Heat exhaustion, or hypovolemia, is the most common condition caused by hot weather exertion. Characteristics include profuse sweating, clammy and cool skin, headache, weakness, nausea, piloerection, rapid pulse, and disorientation. Body temperature is normal. The victim should be removed from the hot environment, undressed, and rehydrated with cool liquids and should rest. Referral is necessary only if symptoms persist.

Frostbite.   Frostbite is freezing of a body part when heat supply inadequately counteracts heat loss. The degree of injury depends on the temperature, wind velocity, time of exposure, humidity, and protective or wet clothing. Symptoms progress from redness and tingling to blanching with no pain. Treatment for first- or second-degree frostbite includes rewarming with breath, a covering, or contact with a warm body area, such as the axilla or a warm water bath (100 to 103°F). Rewarming should continue until the area flushes and tingles. The area should never be rubbed to rewarm; friction may cause more mechanical tissue damage. Alcohol, smoking, and some drugs (marijuana) cause peripheral vasodilatation and blood cooling and are contraindicated. Deep frostbite requires medical attention.

Fractures and Dislocations.   Bone and joint injuries are common in athletics. Any body area can be damaged secondary to a fall, blow, or torque.

The primary basic systems should be evaluated and stabilized. A history should be taken to document the injury mechanism, location and behavior of pain, onset of symptoms (sudden or gradual), previous injury, and specific training procedures or changes. Clothing and equipment should be removed, even if cutting away is necessary. Indications of trauma or hemorrhage, obvious asymmetry, and deformity or abnormal position of a body part should be noted. The area should be palpated to localize the problem and assess sensation and circulation distal to the injury. Specific stress should not be applied if fracture or dislocation is suspected.

Specific signs of a fracture or dislocation include localized point tenderness, decreased functional ability, immediate swelling, obvious deformity or asymmetry, abnormal motion, and instability. All potential fractures and dislocations demand immediate care and referral. Neither injury should be reduced by anyone other than a physician. Reduction may cause neurovascular damage or exacerbation of the fracture or dislocation.

The area should be treated with ice, elevated, and immobilized. Ice reduces cell metabolism, therefore minimizing further damage; edema, by causing vasoconstriction; pain secondary to slow nerve conduction; and muscular activity, by slowing spindle firing. Elevation aids in controlling edema. Immobilization by splinting prevents motion of the injured area, alleviates pain, and reduces further injury. The joint and bone above and below the injury should be immobilized by the splint. All open wounds should be covered and the splint or area padded. The area should be splinted in the current position. A splint or sling and a swathe may be required on shoulder and humeral problems. Pelvic fractures require immobilization on a spine board to prevent additional internal organ injury. A traction splint should be used for femoral fractures. Splints may consist of air-inflation devices, slings, boards, or other implements as necessary. The victim should be referred for immediate care.

Third Priority

Other Musculoskeletal Injuries.   Less serious but more common musculoskeletal injuries in sports include sprains, strains, ruptures, and contusions, which result from falls, blows, torque, and overuse. Immediate attention is required to evaluate the injury accurately and minimize damage. Follow-up evaluation is necessary to determine rehabilitative plans of care and readiness for return to activity.

The assessment plan for a fracture or dislocation injury should be followed for all musculoskeletal injuries. Palpation should be very specific and assess all bone, joint, and soft tissue structures. Joint stability should be assessed. Accurate and thorough assessment defines the structures involved and the severity of the injury. Assessment is most accurate if done immediately, before pain and swelling exacerbate and mask signs.

The management of choice consists of rest, ice application, compression, and elevation. Splinting and the use of crutches may be necessary in more severe injuries. If there is instability, weight-bearing stress should be alleviated and the victim should be referred for radiograph. If the area is stable, sport-specific functional testing should be conducted. Return to activity is indicated only if all symptoms and signs normalize and all functional testing is completed without difficulty.

Sunburn.   Sunburn can occur in any outdoor sport in a hot or cold, high-altitude environment. It is best prevented with sun-blocking agent. Mild to moderate sunburn can be treated with a mild analgesic, ice, or boric acid soaks. More severe burns should be cleansed gently and covered with a dry dressing. Further exposure to sun should be reduced.

Abrasions and Lacerations.   Abrasions, loss of superficial skin layers, and lacerations, wounds secondary to tearing, are frequent in athletic activities and require immediate first aid care.

The area should be evaluated for additional damage. It should be cleansed with soap and water and debris should be removed to prevent infection, then dressed with a nonadhesive pad before return to activity. A special pad or pressure-relief doughnut might be required on some areas for additional protection. Larger abrasions and lacerations may require closure with special bandaging techniques or referral for debridement and suturing. A tetanus injection every 8 years is suggested.

Blisters.   Blisters are caused by skin or mechanical irritation. Fluid in a blister can be clear exudate or blood. The cause and severity of the problem should be determined. Unless very large or functionally deterring, blisters should be allowed to rupture independently. Then the areas should be cleaned, dressed, and protected. Petroleum jelly should be applied over the dressing to reduce further friction.

Bacterial, Fungal, and Viral Skin Lesions.   Because of stress to the organism and development of a moist, warm, and humid environment in many body bacterial, fungal, and viral skin lesions are common in athletes. Aggressive evaluation and care are necessary to prevent self- and team contamination.

The area should be cleansed thoroughly and dressed to prevent infection and further contamination. Appropriate antifungal or antibacterial agents can be used to reduce the severity of the symptoms. Exclusion from team play may be necessary for certain highly contagious conditions, such as impetigo, tinea corporis (ringworm), and herpes.

SUMMARY

Effective and accurate immediate evaluation and management are a vital part of total injury prevention and rehabilitation. This process is more efficient and effective when triage is a part of the plan.

SUGGESTED READINGS

American Red Cross: Standard First Aid and Personal Safety. 2nd Ed. Doubleday and Company, Garden City, New York, 1979

Anderson G, Haycock C, Zydlo S: American Medical Association's Handbook of First Aid and Emergency Care, 1980

Arnheim D: Modern Principles of Athletic Training. 6th Ed. Times Mirror/Mosby Collage Publishing, St. Louis, Missouri, 1985

Bakhaus de Carmo P, Patterson A: First Aid Principles and Procedures. Englewood Cliffs, New Jersey, Prentice Hall, 1976

Birrer R (ed): Sports Medicine for the Primary Care Physician. Appleton–Century–Crafts, Norwalk, Connecticut, 1984

Booker J, Thibodeau G: Athletic Inquiry Assessment. Times Mirror/Mosby–College Publishers, St. Louis, Missouri, 1985

Budassi S: Mosby's Manual of Emergency Care, CV Mosby, St. Louis, Missouri, 1984

Committee on Allied Health, American Academy of Orthopedic Surgeons: Emergency Care and Transportation of the Sick and Injured. 2nd Ed., Chicago, 1977

Donegan J: Cardiopulmonary Resuscitation. Charles C. Thomas, Springfield, Illinois, 1982

Eliastam M, Sternbach C, Bresler M: Manual of Emergency Medicine. 4th Ed. Yearbook Medical Publishers, Chicago, 1983

Erven L: Handbook of Emergency Care and Injuries. Glencoe Press, Beverly Hills, 1976

Gazzan A: Emergency Care: Principles and Practices for the EMT–Paramedic. 2nd Ed. Restow Publishing Company, A Prentice–Hall Company, Reston, Virginia, 1982

Hafen B, Karren K: Prehospital Emergency Care and Crisis Intervention. 2nd Ed. Morton Publishing Company, Englewood, California, 1983

Kuland D: The Injured Athlete. JB Lippincott, Philadelphia, 1982

Marsden N: Diagnosis before First Aid. Churchill Livingstone, Edinburgh, 1978

Parcel G: Basic Emergency Care of the Sick and Injured. 2nd Ed. CV Mosby, St. Louis, Missouri, 1982

Phillips C: Basic Life Support Skills Manual. Robert J. Brady Company, Bowie, Maryland, 1977

Roy S, Irvin R: Sports Medicine. Prentice–Hall, Englewood Cliffs, New Jersey, 1983

Rund D, Rausch T: Triage. CV Mosby, St. Louis, Missouri, 1981

Schneider F: Orthopedics in Emergency Care. CV Mosby, St. Louis, Missouri, 1980

Scott N, Nisonson B, Nicholas J (eds): Principles of Sports Medicine. Williams and Wilkins, Baltimore, 1984

Soper R, MacDonald S, Copass M, Eisenberg M: EMT Manual. WB Saunders, Philadelphia, 1984

Sports Medicine Today Film Series: Examination of the Injured Athlete. Vol. 1, Program 2, 1979

Standards for Cardiopulmonary Resuscitation (CPR) and Emergency Cardiac Care (ECC). JAMA 227:suppl. 7, 1974

Tong J (ed): Athletic Injuries to the Head, Neck and Face. Lea & Febiger, Philadelphia, 1982

Yost C (ed): Sports Safety. AAHPER Division of Safety Education, 1971

8 | Rehabilitation of Sports Injuries: A Practical Approach

John M. Davis

Just as many areas of medicine have become specialties in the past few decades, the evaluation and rehabilitation of sports injuries has become an area of specialization within the profession of physical therapy. Rehabilitation is the physical therapist's bailiwick, and the basic principles of rehabilitation apply whether the patient is an athlete or an elderly person. The long-term goal is to return the patient to a level at which he or she can function as efficiently, effectively, and comfortably as is medically prudent. It is hoped that the patient will return to "normal," with the realization that normal is a subjective term. For the elderly person, normal may mean accomplishing simple domestic tasks without experiencing pain and weakness. Following successful therapy, this person would be able to walk, garden, cook, and perform other low-intensity activities without difficulty. The same basic goals apply to the athlete, but once the athlete can perform low-intensity activities, the emphasis should shift to high-intensity activities and movement demanded in sport. This is crucial before the athlete can return to competition. The athlete desires to perform activities of daily living comfortably and effectively, but his or her normal activities may include colliding with a 250-pound lineman or sprinting at breakneck speed. Therefore the therapist directing the athlete's rehabilitation must take into account the stresses that the athlete's sport will place upon him or her and work toward reconditioning the athlete so that his or her physical capabilities on return to competition will match the demands of the activity.

The physical therapist is uniquely trained to handle this client. The therapist's education includes the etiology of athletic injury, the physiology of athletic endeavor, the principles of first aid, the theories of joint motion, and the theories of strength training. Numerous sources are available on developing an effective program of therapeutic exercise for the injured athlete. Journals, texts, and short courses by the American Physical Therapy Association, the National Athletic Trainers Association, and various orthopaedic groups are excellent resources.

THE ATHLETE AND HIS OR HER ENTOURAGE

In dealing with athletes, the therapist will come into contact with many people who have an interest in the athlete's well-being. The therapist needs to develop a rapport with the athlete and some members of the entourage: the physician, the family, the team trainer, and the coach. He or she may be called upon by the media, professional sports teams, agents, and gamblers to provide information concerning the athlete's health. These groups should be approached with professionalism.

Athletes' basic health is generally good, and medical complications are rare. As a rule they are highly motivated and will cooperate enthusiastically in a rehabilitation program. The therapist must develop a strong rapport with the athlete. Athletes are accustomed to following instructions from a well-trained person, the coach, and are more likely to trust and follow the recommendations of the therapist if he or she is confident and efficient. Athletes are sensitive to wasted time and effort—they are accustomed to producing maximum effort and expect the same from their team. During the rehabilitation process, the therapist becomes a crucial part of the team. The therapist must devote maximum effort to the athlete's rehabilitation.

As a member of the team, the therapist may experience some unusual demands: treatments early or late in the day and on weekends, late night telephone calls, and other stresses on time and patience. But if the therapist wishes to become respected by the athletic community and to develop a close and rewarding rapport with the athlete, he must be both flexible and willing to make extra effort a part of the treatment plan. Often a fine line separates acceptable competitive performance from the danger of reinjury. The therapist who is closely attuned with the athlete will offer better judgment regarding the athlete's ability to perform safely and effectively.

Usually the athlete is referred for therapy by a physician, maybe the team physician who is closely involved in providing comprehensive medical care for the athlete, or maybe a physician who has little experience in the care of sports injuries and who is less available for consultation. The therapist must determine the extent of the physician's involvement in the rehabilitative process and plan accordingly. The therapist may be given a very detailed referral and rehabilitation protocol by a team physician and be expected to follow it closely or may be told simply to evaluate and treat, allowing the therapist a free hand.

Ideally, the physician will be interested and involved in the rehabilitation process. When the therapist and physician develop a good professional relationship, decisionmaking can be a cooperative effort. The therapist spends a great amount of time with the athlete, both treating and reassessing progress, and hence develops an insight into the progress and problems of the client that can be most helpful to the physician. As the physician monitors the successful progress of the client, his or her trust in the therapist's knowledge and ability increases. Thus the rehabilitative process becomes a true team effort.

The injury of a family member can cause reactions within the family ranging from disinterest to support to hostility toward the rehabilitative effort. The therapist spends a vast amount of time with the client during rehabilitation, so he or she may be viewed as the most accessible health professional. The therapist should treat the family with respect and should answer questions truthfully and discreetly. All information should coincide with the opinion of the referring physician; if the therapist is in disagreement with the physician, the conflict should be resolved before an opinion is expressed to a family member. When the family members trust the physician and the therapist, they will be more inclined to cooperate with the rehabilitation program; they will supervise the home program and report any problems that the patient may be reluctant to admit. The family can be either the greatest resource available or one of the greatest hindrances during rehabilitation.

Parents may pressure the athlete and therapist for a return to competition before the athlete is ready. This may occur for many reasons: money, pride, past experience, or fear of failure. Occasionally parents may try to delay the rehabilitation process to prevent their child from returning to competition because they think athletics are too dangerous for their child. The therapist must be aware of such issues and help to resolve them, still maintaining the rehabilitation effort. It is hoped that the dynamics of the family will aid the recovery of the athlete and that the therapist will be able to recruit family members to help in the rehabilitation process.

Therapists must exercise caution if they are providing care to athletes under the age of consent. Permission from the parent to provide care is necessary before the therapist initiates a treatment. This is important in a school or community setting.

The relationship between the coach and the therapist merits some discussion. Both desire the rapid return of the injured athlete to competition, yet often an adversarial relationship develops between them. It is often best to heed the cliché "Doctors don't coach and coaches don't doctor." This approach must be moderated by common sense. Many coaches realize that they are not trained to treat injuries and welcome assistance in caring for their injured charges. The coach can provide helpful information concerning the etiology of injury and the personality of the athlete. He or she can encourage the rehabilitation process by enforcing exercise programs and training rules. If a good relationship is developed between the coach, the athlete, and the health care team, the rehabilitation effort will be enhanced. The therapist should never allow pressure from the coach to interfere with the objective decision concerning readiness for return to competition. The athlete's health is paramount, so the therapist must ignore any pressure to return the athlete to activity before rehabilitation is completed.

Often, especially if the athlete is a member of a school or professional team, a trainer is a member of the health care team that provides comprehensive medical care for the athlete. Modern athletic trainers are well trained: the National Athletic Trainer's Association has developed a system of certification that ensures that athletic trainers are college graduates who have completed a course of study that resembles the basic science program required of physical therapy students, including the study of athletic injuries and their treatment. Many of these trainers are well-versed in the rehabilitation of athletic injuries and can be a valuable resource for the therapist.

The athletic trainer has a unique position in the rehabilitation process in that he or she usually is present at the beginning and at the end of the process. The trainer is probably the first health care professional to see the athlete following injury, and it is his or her evaluation and first aid that initiates the athlete's journey through the health care system. As the athlete begins to recover, the trainer is best able to observe the patient's progress through various functional activities on the field or court and can provide any protective devices or taping needed prior to activity. It is not possible or practical for the therapist or physician to observe the athlete daily at practice, but the trainer is on the practice field and is trained to provide services to the athlete that will enhance recovery.

The therapist, physician, family, coach, and trainer all have legitimate concerns for the health and condition of the injured athlete. Any information concerning the status of the injured athlete is confidential and must be protected by the health professional. If the injured person is well-known, the therapist may be pressured by the media, friends, and others to divulge information, but the patient's consent, giving this information is a violation of medical confidentiality, and the therapist would be subject to legal censor. When in doubt, silence is the best answer to such inquiries.

It is wise to devise a system of reporting the injured athlete's status to the media. One person should be responsible for drafting a statement, having the statement cleared, and releasing it to the media. Any inquiries concerning the status of the injured person should be referred to this spokesperson.

The therapist may be contacted by professional sports teams or their agents concerning an athlete that the therapist has treated. This information is confidential and cannot be released without written permission from the athlete. Even when such permission is given, the therapist should exercise extreme caution in replying to any questions that require a subjective opinion. The therapist best serves the athlete and the professional organization requesting the information by providing only objective answers.

THE REHABILITATIVE PROCESS

The rehabilitation of an injured athlete begins immediately following the incident with the application of appropriate first aid. An individual trained in first aid should be present at the sporting event or practice. The primary goal of first aid is to cause no further harm, and expediency is crucial only if a life-threatening situation exists. If adequate personnel, equipment, or knowledge is not available to handle the situation properly, it is best to wait until such resources arrive at the scene.

Most athletic injuries are orthopedic in nature and involve the limbs. The best initial treatment for these injuries is rest, ice, compression, and elevation. Rest can be provided to an injured lower extremity by splints and crutches. A sling, swathe, and splints prevent movement and provide for an injured upper extremity. Ice can be provided by chemical packs, plastic ice bags, ice cups, or other cooling techniques. Initially, ice should be applied for 15 to 20 minutes and repeated at frequent intervals during the first 24 hours after injury. Compression is applied with elastic wraps and compressive dressings. The wrapping must not be too snug, because circulation can be impaired. The injured part should be elevated so that it is higher than the heart.

The therapist usually becomes part of the rehabilitation process following the athlete's initial visit to his or her physician. The therapist should strive to produce a spirit of rapport and cooperation with the athlete during the initial meeting. In the first session, the therapist should evaluate the athlete's level of function and dysfunction and document this base-line information for use in program planning and future evaluations.

Using the information from the evaluation, the therapist devises the treatment goals. The short-term goals should include the accomplishment of component skills needed to reach the long-term goal: the return to athletic competition.[1] Unless a condition exists that will prevent full function, the athlete expects to return to his or her sport.

Once the goals are established, a plan of treatment is devised. The plan should work steadily and gradually toward accomplishing the successive short-term goals. It should be flexible: if one approach is not working, the problem should be reevaluated and a new plan devised.

During the rehabilitative process, the emphasis of the treatment plan shifts as certain short-term goals are met. The initial emphasis of the program is on the maintainence of cardiovascular fitness; this remains a major portion of the program until the athlete returns to competition. Also, the return of flexibility and normal range of motion are emphasized. Later, the main thrust of the program shifts to the reestablishment of normal strength and endurance. Eventually the emphasis of the program moves to the resumption of purposeful controlled movement in the athletic setting.[2,3] The therapist must select appropriate modalities and exercises for the program. The tasks and demands placed upon the athlete should be within his or her ability to achieve, providing positive feedback and enhancing compliance with the program. Periodic reevaluation of the patient's progress is essential: once a short-term goal is met, time is wasted if that portion of the program is repeated without augmentation by new goals and activities.

Athletic competition places extreme mental and physical pressure upon the athlete. For the injured athlete to return successfully to competition, he or she must possess normal flexibility, highly developed strength and endurance, excellent cardiovascular conditioning, and the ability to move quickly, forcefully, and purposefully. Because the rehabilitation process must prepare the athlete for such stress, portions of the rehabilitation program must be quite strenuous. The purpose of the rehabilitation program is to allow a return to competition that is safe, with chance of injury minimized.

MODALITIES

Therapeutic modalities such as heat, cold, electricity, light, and sound are all useful parts of the treatment plan. Unfortunately, the various machines and devices employed in the treatment of athletes are sometimes viewed as "get-well machines" that possess magical properties. An athlete may feel slighted if his or her daily treatment does not include a dose of ultrasound, electrical stimulation, laser enlightenment, and some of the popular combinations of blinking lights and clanging bells. The therapist should select the appropriate modality based on a knowledge of the agents' therapeutic properties, not the latest fad.

Modalities are an effective part of the rehabilitation program, but they are just that—a part of the whole. The modality should not be the sole treatment. Physical agents are effective in the early stages of treatment to aid in the reduction of swelling, to reduce pain, to retard muscle atrophy, and to decrease inflammation. However, therapeutic exercise is the most important modality available for the reconditioning of the injured athlete.[4] The long-term goal of the process—the return of motion, strength and endurance, and function—cannot be reached through the use of physical agents alone. Therapeutic exercise is essential and should be initiated as soon as the condition of the athlete allows.

When the selection of modalities is limited, the use of ice, elevation, and manual resistive exercise should not be overlooked. Many conditions can be treated effectively with ice and a skilled therapist's hands. Ice and elevation are quite effective for moderating pain and swelling, and a well-trained therapist can provide effective therapeutic exercise with a minimum of equipment.

DECONDITIONING

Following any but the most trivial injury, the athlete will undergo a period of decreased activity (rest). This period may be as short as 24 hours, following a minor sprain, or as long as 12 months, following a catastrophic knee injury and surgery. As a consequence of this limited activity, systems within the athlete's body undergo changes that result in an overall state of decreased physical fitness, the extent of which is related to the length and nature of the athlete's inactivity and previous level of activity. Research on the deconditioning phenomena by NASA during the Gemini, Apollo, and Skylab missions and Soviet data accumulated during the Vostok and Soyuz flights have documented the effects of long-term inactivity. This research has shown that the cardiovascular, musculoskeletal, and thermoregulatory systems are profoundly affected by forced inactivity.[5]

Research involving the astronauts and healthy volunteers has demonstrated that following inactivity the ability to perform physical work is decreased. Submaximal physical effort causes a higher heart rate, lower stroke volume, and lower cardiac output, resulting in a decreased maximum oxygen consumption.[5] When an individual is placed on forced bedrest or in zero gravity, 600 to 700 ml of blood moves from the legs to the thoracic cavity, causing an increase in central blood volume. This increase sets off a chain reaction that results in peripheral vasodilatation, inhibition of antidiuretic hormone, increased renal blood flow, and inhibition of the release of renin and aldosterone.[5] The result is water diuresis and a decrease in plasma volume. Accompanying this decrease is the development of orthostatic hypotension, the inability of the blood pressure to adjust to a change in posture. When a deconditioned person is suddenly moved from recumbency to standing, approximately 500 ml of blood moves quickly from the thorax to the legs. As a result of this movement of blood and the already-depleted plasma volume, the cardiac output and blood pressure decrease and the amount of blood traveling to the brain drops.[5] This manifests an increased heart rate, sweating, pallor, and possible syncope.

Deossification of weight-bearing bones has been noted following prolonged rest or cast immobilization. This occurs independent of calcium intake; demineralization of the os calcis has been found within days of immobilization.[5] The deossification is due to the lack of weightbearing; only pressure applied through the longitudinal axis of the bone reverses the process.

A loss of muscle strength and bulk likewise has been noted following prolonged rest. Nitrogen excretion in the urine increases during inactivity and reaches a maximum by the 10th day.[5] The increase in nitrogen excretion is related to a reduced protein synthesis rather than a breakdown of existing tissue. Since the immobilized part cannot be exercised, the muscles of that area are not stressed; without stress there is no feedback to indicate that the muscles need protein for rebuilding. The increase in nitrogen indicates that the muscles are deteriorating and that muscle mass and strength are decreasing. Increased uptake of protein does not change the deterioration; only resisted movement of the affected area has an effect.

Thermoregulation is adversely altered by inactivity. Although the exact mechanism for the change is unclear, it is thought to be related to the decrease in blood plasma volume. During work, the core temperature of volunteers placed on bedrest rose more rapidly, rose to a higher level, and took longer to return to normal than the core temperature of healthy subjects. Also, sweating occurred more easily and at a lower skin temperature in the group on forced bedrest.[5]

The crews of the more recent space flights have combatted deconditioning very effectively by following a regular regimen of physical activity. They used bicycle ergometers and treadmills to maintain cardiovascular fitness and inflatable trousers to prevent a decrease in blood pressure. They performed resistance exercises for the major muscle groups using pulleys, weights, and springs or isometric exercises if equipment was unavailable. Longitudinal pressure to the axis of the long bones was applied with a spring-loaded device. A similar device has been developed for hospital use to prevent deossification in the bones of bedridden patients.

Deconditioning can be devastating to the athlete. It can lead to demoralization and a delayed return to competition. The rehabilitation program must attack this problem from the outset. The therapist should incorporate into the initial program activities that combat the deconditioning process. It is much easier to maintain fitness than to recondition the athlete.

When feasible, early mobilization and weightbearing are desirable to prevent deossification of the weight-bearing bones. It is usually easy to incorporate some type of aerobic activity into the exercise program for cardiovascular maintainence. Walking, jogging, cycling, swimming, and other activities that require prolonged repetitive use of the body's large muscle groups are an excellent means of maintaining cardiovascular fitness. To maintain fitness, the intensity of the activity should demand 50 to 70 percent of maximum oxygen.[5,6] This roughly corresponds to a heart rate within the range of 65 to 75 percent of the predicted maximum heart rate. The maximum heart rate (HRMAX) and maximum oxygen consumption can be calculated with a treadmill stress test or predicted by the formula:

$$\text{HRMAX} = 210 - (\text{age} \times 0.65)$$

The workout should be 20 to 30 minutes long, three to five times per week. [5,6] Such an exercise regimen will maintain the cardiovascular status; increasing the parameters of the program should improve aerobic fitness. The presence of heart disease should be ascertained before an older athlete begins such a program.

General strengthening exercises for the uninvolved parts of the athlete's body should be performed three to five times per week.[5,7] The exercises can be isometric, isotonic, or isokinetic, but they should be sufficient to maintain the athlete's current level of strength. When possible, isometric exercises and electrical stimulation should be used on the muscles of an immobilized limb.

FLEXIBILITY

In sports medicine, flexibility refers to two different phenomena: the flexibility that results from training for a certain athletic event, which may be well beyond what is considered normal range of motion (ROM); and the lack of flexibility that results from an injury. Flexibility is the combined result of the condition of the soft tissues that surround a joint. The joint configuration may limit the end points of motion. The condition of the ligaments, tendons, joint capsule, and muscles also affect flexibility. Flexibility is related to age, sex, and activity level. Generally, young, active people (especially women) are more flexible. Some athletic movements, such as gymnastics, pitching, and dancing require an abnormal amount of flexibility: the therapist must account for this in the treatment program. Maintenance of good flexibility allows an athlete to compete comfortably with a decreased risk of injury.[8,9]

Lack of flexibility and ROM resulting from an injury are the problems likely to be seen in a clinic. Any trauma to the soft tissues surrounding a joint can restrict motion. Therefore, damage to the articular cartilage, synovium, joint capsule, muscle, ligament, or tendon of a joint can hinder movements significantly. Damage to any of these structures will cause inflammation and swelling. Rupture of a capsule, ligament, and/or tendon may result in joint instability. To complicate further the loss of motion, the initial injury may be followed by the trauma of a surgical procedure.

Following surgery or prolonged immobilization, a lack of motion is secondary to either capsular or ligamentous shortening.[10] A synovial effusion may be another cause of decreased motion and should be managed before effective motion can be restored. In the case of surgery, tightening of the joint capsule may have been the aim of the procedure, so caution must be exercised in regaining the lost motion.

The ligaments and capsule form the static supports of the joint and are composed of fibroblasts lined in rows parallel to the collagen fibers. The collagen fibers run parallel to the axis of tension placed on the joint. A ground substance made of water and protoglycons forms an extracellular matrix that separates the collagen fibers, allowing them to elongate to their maximum. When pathological shortening occurs, this ground substance is lost and the buffer between the collagen fibers weakened.[10] Crosslinkage between the fibers occurs and the elongation of the fibers is decreased. To reverse this process, the ground substance must be restored and the crosslinkages between the fibers ruptured. Many techniques have been used to correct this shortening: active motion of antagonist muscles, prolonged passive stretch at low force, temperature elevation of the shortened structures during prolonged low-force stretch, and various mobilization techniques that emphasize the normal gliding motion of the affected joint.[10] In severe cases, serial casting and manipulation under anesthesia are required to regain normal ROM.

Muscle contracture also can cause a decrease in motion, but fortunately this does not cause a major problem in the treatment of athletic injuries. A muscle contracture occurs when, on elongation, the muscle is not long enough to produce a full ROM. This is believed to occur as a result of changes either in the length at the origin or insertional aponeurosis of the muscle or in muscle fiber length.[10] It is often difficult to ascertain whether motion is decreased by capsular shortening or muscle contracture. In sports medicine, an individual joint is rarely immobilized long enough to cause a severe muscle contracture. Muscle contractures respond very slowly. Short-term stretch is ineffective; serial casting or surgery may be needed to correct a severe problem.[10]

STRENGTH AND ENDURANCE

When the athlete approaches normal ROM in the injured joint, the emphasis of the rehabilitation should shift from flexibility to exercises that enhance the strength of the muscles surrounding the injured area. Flexibility remains an important aspect of the total program, but strength-training exercises are introduced with great frequency and intensity. Initially, manual-resistive and isometric exercises should be used and can be incorporated into the flexibility program. As the athlete becomes stronger, more strenuous resistive exercises should be introduced.

There are three basic types of resistive exercise: isometric, isotonic, and isokinetic. In recent years the equipment used to provide these types of resistance has become increasingly sophisticated. Therapeutic exercise has moved from the cast-iron weight boot to the computerized isokinetic devices of the 1980s. Still, the basic principle of strength improvement remains the same: to increase strength, the muscle must be stressed to the point of overload.[2,3,7,11,12] The overload can be provided manually or by machine. The effectiveness of manual resistance should not be overlooked: it can enhance strength gain greatly when employed in conjunction with proprioceptive neuromuscular facilitation patterns and functional movements. It is also very useful both early in the strength-gaining process, when only minimal amounts of resistance can be tolerated, and late in the process, when various motions require fine tuning.

Many of the new sophisticated pieces of exercise equipment are quite effective and useful in rehabilitation, but the equipment is only as good as the therapist who designs and supervises the exercise program. Safe, purposeful, and specific resistance is the key to strength gain. The choice of method for providing resistance must be made by the therapist based on affordability of the equipment, practicality of the exercise, and safety.

Three principles must be followed to ensure a gain in strength: overload, gradual progression, and specificity. The muscle must be stressed to the point of overload (the work required of the muscle must be greater than the work normally required of the muscle.) As the muscle becomes stronger, the amount of stress required to produce overload increases; therefore, the amount of resistance provided during exercise must increase. This increase must follow a gradual progression so that the exercise remains comfortable and safe. Finally, the exercise must be specific; to strengthen a specific muscle that muscle must be isolated so the bulk of the resistance falls upon it.[2,6,7,13] Regardless of the type of equipment use in the rehabilitation program, if a specific muscle is provided a gradually progressing overloading resistance, strength and endurance will increase.

TYPE OF EXERCISE

Isometric

During an isometric contraction, the muscle contracts and the muscle belly increases in size, but there is no joint motion or functional movement. The muscle produces a force equal to the resistance provided. Isometric exercises are useful when ROM is limited by injury or casting. Brief repetitive isometric maximal exercise (BRIME) has been shown to be an effective means of increasing strength when the exercise is performed with a 6-second maximal isometric contraction followed by a 20-second rest. This procedure should be repeated 20 times per day.[14]

Advantages. The advantages of isometric exercises are

Little or no equipment is required;
There is little danger of causing joint irritation;
It can be performed on any muscle;
Neural associations are maintained through muscle contractions that stimulate the mechanoreceptor system in the joint capsule and surrounding ligaments and tendons;
Muscle atrophy in immobilized limbs is retarded.[9,14,15]

Disadvantages. The disadvantages of isometric exercises are

Strength increases are specifically at the angle of the joint during exercise;
There is no positive feedback and little patient motivation;
Muscular endurance is not enhanced;
Eccentric contractions do not occur;
The blood pressure can increase if the length of the contraction is greater than 6 seconds or the rest between contractions less than 20 seconds.[9,14,15]

Isotonic

An isotonic muscle contraction occurs when the muscle either shortens or lengthens, joint motion occurs, and work is performed. The contraction is a concentric isotonic contraction if the muscle shortens during the contraction and an eccentric isotonic contraction if the muscle lengthens during the contraction. In an isotonic exercise, the prime mover performs a concentric contraction (the biceps femoris causes knee flexion) followed by an eccentric contraction (the biceps femoris controls the weight of the lower leg as the knee moves from flexion to extension). Eccentric contractions are an excellent means of increasing muscular tension but are the primary cause of residual muscular soreness.[15] This soreness can lead to decreased performance secondary to pain and biochemical changes in the muscle. Eccentric contractions are useful early in the rehabilitation process, when concentric contractions may not be possible to perform. Because many functional activities require eccentric contractions, they should be included in the program.

Isotonic exercises can be divided further into constant-resistance and variable-resistance exercises. Constant resistance is the classic type of isotonic exercise: the dumbell is raised, the free weight is bench-pressed, and the weight boot is taken from flexion to extension. The resistance does not change during exercise, so the amount of weight that can be employed must correspond to the weakest point in the ROM. Variable resistance is possible when commercially manufactured devices are used. These machines are engineered with either a cam system (Nautilus, Eagle) or a changing lever arm length (Universal) so that the resistance varies through the join ROM. In theory, the device should provide less resistance at the weak points in the range and greater resistance at the strong points; however, the engineering has been questioned. The devices that employ a cam system supposedly provide resistance equal to the normal strength curve of the muscle being exercised, but individuals have varying limb and muscle lengths, so exercise is not truly customized.[15] The machines that incorporate a changing lever arm length do not take into account the velocity by which most of the work occurs early in the ROM.[15] This is not to imply that these machines are poorly designed or faulty. On the contrary, they provide an excellent means of isotonic resistance. The theories behind the development of these machines are as new as the devices themselves and should be examined closely. The machines are being improved constantly and are a reasonable part of a well-rounded strength training program.

Isotonic exercise regimes vary. The DeLorme progressive resistive exercise (PRE) program of 3 sets of 10 repetitions at 50 percent, 75 percent, and 100 percent of maximum contraction is the oldest of all isotonic programs.[7,11] The variables that can be adjusted in isotonic exercise include the number of sets, the number of repetitions per set, the amount and progression of resistance, and the frequency of exercise by day and by week. Since the number of variables is high, the number of variations is great also. Generally, isotonic exercise is performed in repetitive sets of 8 to 12 repetitions a minimum of 3 to 5 times per week. As long as the principles of overload, specificity, and gradual progression are followed in a program customized to the specific needs of the athlete, strength will increase.

Advantages.   The advantages of isotonic exercise are

Strength develops throughout the entire ROM;
Endurance is enhanced;
Muscle size increases;
Some of the equipment is inexpensive and easy to use;
Motivation increases with improvement;
Exercise is both concentric and eccentric.[7,9,15]

Disadvantages.   The disadvantages of isotonic exercise are

Equipment can be expensive and require large amounts of space;
The amount of weight employed may be limited by the weakest point in the ROM;
Momentum decreases the effectiveness of the exercise;

The device exercises only one muscle group;

Traumatic synovitis can occur if the overload is excessive;

Danger can result if there is pain during movement because the limb must continue supporting the weight;

Exercise does not occur at functional speeds.[7,9,15]

Isokinetic

Isokinetic exercise is the newest form of resistive exercise and still is being refined. Developed by James Perrine in the late 1960s, the theory of isokinetics is to provide exercise at a dynamic preset speed with a resistance that accommodates throughout the entire ROM.[15] The implications for the use of isokinetics are great. Coupled with computer technology, isokinetics is changing the conventional methods of strength training.

The devices employed to provide isokinetic resistance (e.g., Cybex, Orthotron, Kin-Com) are becoming progressively more sophisticated and complicated. Essentially, they are designed to provide a lever that can be moved at a preset speed. The preset speed remains constant, but the resistance varies and matches the force applied on the lever. Therefore the resistance is accommodating; the design of the device allows for maximum resistance at each point within the range of motion. This theory is a great departure from isometric and isotonic exercise because muscles can be overloaded at every point in the ROM and the speeds of the exercise are much closer to the limb speeds encountered during functional activities.[15]

The development of isokinetic exercise regimes is an ongoing process, still very much experimental and open to modification. Many programs recommend the use of timed exercise sets, opposed to the number of repetitions per set parameters in isotonic programs. Most isokinetic programs are based on the principles and programs described by Davies.[15]

Advantages. The advantages of isokinetic exercise are

The muscle receives maximum overload throughout the ROM;

Exercise is safe because resistance stops with the cessation of motion;

Resistance accommodates to the weaker points in the ROM;

Decreased joint compression occurs at higher speeds;

Training can be done at varying speeds;

The patient can receive immediate feedback;

Objective data can be gathered for patient evaluation.[9,13,15]

Disadvantages. The disadvantages of isokinetic exercise are

Equipment is expensive;

No eccentric contraction occurs;

Equipment attachments are cumbersome and inconvenient to adjust;

Equipment breakdown and servicing needs are frequent;

Personnel must be trained in equipment use and interpretation of data.[9,13,15]

Muscular Endurance

It is difficult to separate the development of strength from the development of endurance; both occur simultaneously, one outdistancing the other depending on the emphasis of the exercise program. Classically isometric exercises are viewed as poor developers of muscular endurance.[9] On the other hand, isotonics and isokinetics both increase endurance. As the strength development portion of the rehabilitation reaches a maximum, the emphasis shifts to endurance training, although the process of strength training and general conditioning provide a degree of endurance training. This phase consists of fine tuning and refining the endurance already developed. With isotonic exercise, muscular endurance is increased by increasing the number of repetitions within a given set or by increasing the number of sets. With isokinetics, endurance can be enhanced by increasing the length (time) of each exercise bout. Generally, endurance is increased by working against a submaximal resistance in a highly repetitious manner. Many functional activities are excellent for providing this type of exercise and should be incorporated into the exercise program.

Functional Activity

Functional activities are emphasized in the next phase of the rehabilitation program. Some functional activities were probably initiated as part of a general conditioning program (e.g., swimming, cycling), but more specific exercises are introduced to enhance proprioception, coordination, mobility, flexibility, strength, and endurance. These activities should mimic the component motions of the sport as closely as possible.

Functional activities for the upper extremity might include manually or isokinetically resisted PNF patterns, isotonically resisted diagonals, wall pully exercises through specific motions, resisted movement via rubber tubing, swimming, upper extremity cycling, or other facsimiles of the athletic activity. For the lower extremity, resisted PNF patterns, bicycling, trampolining, lateral step-ups, rope jumping, and other imaginative exercises can be used to provide a functional stress to the injured area in a safely guarded manner. With gradual exposure of the injured part to the stress of the sport, the shock of return to high-intensity movement can be dampened. When the athlete can perform the component motions of the sport safely and effectively, the actual motions of the sport are resumed; the basketball player recovering from an ankle sprain would progress from trampolining to rope jumping to flat-footed jumping to a jump-shot. These are resumed at a low level of intensity and gradually increased.

Deciding when the injured athlete can return to full participation in his or her sport can be difficult. The decision requires a thorough evaluation of the athlete. In addition to objective data, the examiner's subjective perception of the athlete's ability to perform safely in a dangerous situation is used to reach a decision.

When the athlete has reached what objectively appears to be the end of the rehabilitation, certain criteria must be met before he or she can be allowed to resume competition. The injured area should be free of pain with no evidence of swelling and should have normal ROM and normal strength. Strength can be tested isokinetically, by comparing torque values of the injured limb with the opposite extremity or with a previous test of the involved extremity if the test was prior to the injury, or isotonically by comparing the maximum amount of weight that can be moved by one limb with that of the other. Appropriate functional tests must be completed without evidence of disability. The functional testing should be assessed by a knowledgeable individual, preferably the physician, therapist, or trainer. The coach has an understandable conflict of interest and should not be the sole judge of functional ability. For the lower extremity, these functional tests should include but not be limited to full-speed sprinting and cutting, running progressively smaller figure eights, one-leg hopping, and other motions involved in a particular sport. If there is limping, swelling, or pain, the athlete has failed the test. For the upper extremity, the tests might include progressively longer and harder throwing or passing, repeated and varying amounts of manual resistance to the motion in question, and other activity-appropriate tests. Pain, apprehension, and swelling are cause for disqualification. The decision to allow the resumption of activity must be based on performance also. Even if the objective data indicate that the athlete is ready for action, he or she must be disqualified if his or her performance of the functional tests appears impaired.

Once the decision to allow the athlete to resume competition has been made, protective taping and bracing should be considered. Although taping joints for protection during athletics has been done for many years, the effectiveness is questionable. The application of the tape requires fine motor training but can be learned with practice. Some institutions and professional teams require every team member to have his or her ankles taped before each practice and game. This is quite an expense for a procedure that may be of little value. The debate over the effectiveness of ankle taping is as old as the practice itself and is yet to be resolved. I agree with the conclusions stated by Emerich[16]: (1) taping loses supporting strength during exercise; (2) individuals whose ankles are taped are less likely to injure their ankles than those whose ankles are untaped; (3) taping may stimulate muscle action rather than weaken ankle musculature; and (4) taping the ankle does not place the knee in greater jeopardy for injury. Tape should never be used on any injured joint unless a proper rehabilitation program has been instituted. Tape is not a substitute for exercise.

Two types of knee braces are receiving a great amount of use and attention in athletic and medical circles. One type is designed to prevent knee injury (Omni, MacDavid, Don Joy) and the other is designed to protect the injured knee, especially from rotatory stress (Lenox Hill, Pro Am). At a recent meeting, the Committee for Sports Medicine of the American Academy of Orthopaedic Surgeons noted that basic research on the design and function of these braces was lacking (T. Taft, personal communication). Some limited studies have been completed, but the data are sparse considering the large number of braces in use. This is not to imply that these braces are faulty—further research may show them to be quite functional and effective—but until more information is available, the choice of such a brace is a matter of personal preference, based on past experience and physician recommendation. Bracing should always augment, not replace, a sound rehabilitation program.

SUMMARY

Physical therapy has gradually specialized over the past few decades. Just as other patient populations have been recognized as having special needs, so has the population of athletes. Although injured athletes have unique problems, the basic principles of rehabilitation apply to their treatment.

The rehabilitation process begins with adequate first aid for the injury; this should limit the extent of the injury and hasten the return of function. Following a thorough evaluation of the athlete and the injury, the therapist devises and institutes a rehabilitation program that progressively emphasizes the return of normal ROM, the maintenance of cardiovascular conditioning, the retardation of muscular atrophy, the return of normal strength and endurance, and, at the appropriate time, functional activities that stimulate the return of coordinated and purposeful movement. The progress of the athlete should be evaluated at regular intervals during the rehabilitation process and the program adjusted as indicated. When the athlete reaches the point in the program at which he or she is ready to resume full activity, he or she must pass performance tests. If the tests are completed successfully and if the objective data from the evaluation are indicative of normal function, the athlete is allowed to resume activity.

REFERENCES

1. O'Sullivan S, Cullen K, Schitz T: Physical Rehabilitation, FA Davis, Philadelphia, 1981
2. Aten D, Knight K: Therapeutic exercise in athletic training: principles and overview. Athletic Training, 13:123, 1978.
3. Houglum P: The modality of therapeutic exercise: objectives and principles. Athletic Training, 12:42, 1977
4. Ruskin A: Current Therapy in Physiatry. WB Saunders, Philadelphia, 1981
5. Kavanagh T: General deconditioning. p. 237. In Medical Rehabilitation. Williams and Wilkins, Baltimore, 1984
6. Cooper K: The Aerobics Way. M Evans, New York, 1977
7. de Lateur B: Exercise for strength and endurance. p. 86. In Therapeutic Exercise. 3rd Ed. Williams and Wilkins, Baltimore, 1978

8. Boland A: Rehabilitation of the injured athlete. p. 226. In Sports Medicine and Physiology. WB Saunders, Philadelphia, 1979
9. Miller D, Allen T: Fitness: A Lifetime Commitment. Burgess, Minneapolis, 1982
10. Stolov W: Mobility problems of the muscle–joint unit. p. 196. In Medical Rehabilitation. Williams and Wilkins, Baltimore, 1984
11. Allman F: Exercise in sports medicine. p. 450. In Therapeutic Exercise. 3rd Ed. Williams and Wilkins, Baltimore, 1978
12. Knuttgen H: Physical conditioning and limits to performance. p. 94. In Sports Medicine and Physiology. WB Saunders, Philadelphia, 1979
13. Cooper M, Adrian M, Glassow R: Kinesiology. p. 380. CV Mosby, St. Louis, 1982
14. Liberson W: Brief isometric exercises. p. 201. In Therapeutic Exercise. 3rd Ed. Williams and Wilkins, Baltimore, 1978
15. Davies G: A Compendium of Isokinetics in Clinical Usage. S & S Publishers, LaCrosse, Wisconsin, 1984
16. Emerich C: Ankle taping: prevention of injury or waste of time. Athletic Training, 14:49, 1979

SUGGESTED READINGS

Books

Hoppenfeld S: Physical Examination of the Spine and Extremities. Appleton–Century–Crofts, New York, 1976

Kessler R, Hertling D: Management of Common Musculoskeletal Disorders. Harper and Row, Philadelphia, 1983

Roy W, Irvin R: Sports Medicine: Prevention, Evaluation, Management, and Rehabilitation, Prentice–Hall, Englewood Cliffs, New Jersey, 1983

Journals

The American Journal of Sports Medicine, The American Orthopaedic Society for Sports Medicine, Williams and Wilkins Publisher, Baltimore

Athletic Training, The National Athletic Trainer's Association, Greenville, North Carolina

The Journal of Orthopaedic and Sports Physical Therapy, The American Physical Therapy Association-Orthopaedic and Sports Medicine Sections, Williams and Wilkins Publisher, Baltimore

9 | Psychology of Sports and the Injured Athlete

David Yukelson

During the past two decades, the area of sports psychology has emerged as a reputable and legitimate field of scientific inquiry that is recognized and appreciated by athletes, coaches, physicians, physical therapists, and athletic trainers as an integral discipline within sports medicine. Unlike general psychotherapy, which deals with individuals who have profound and often deepseated psychological problems, sports psychology is concerned with understanding why people in sports behave as they do. For instance, why do some athletes rise to the challenge when their best efforts are most needed while others seem to fall apart when the going gets tough? Why do some athletes bounce back from a debilitating injury very quickly with a sense of pride, confidence, and renewed determination to get better while others appear to wallow in self-pity for prolonged periods of time and never really realize their potential capabilities? What actions on the part of an athletic trainer or physical therapist motivate or discourage athletes in their quest for rehabilitating themselves from an athletic injury?

In essence, sports psychology looks at the influence that sports participation has on the psyche of the sports enthusiast in terms of personality development, attitude formation, anxiety reduction, and psychological wellbeing. In addition, it looks at the effect of psychological variables, such as motivation, confidence, concentration, emotional self-control, and various interpersonal relationships, on performance.[1] Through scientific inquiry (i.e., theoretical and applied research), sports psychologists test their suppositions about how psychological factors influence sports performance and how sports participation may influence the athletes' psychological development and personal growth.

Although the area of sports psychology is diverse, its objective is relatively simple: to optimize competence and self-respect in athletes through the development of psychological skills training programs that enable them to perform better and gain maximal satisfaction from their efforts.[2] Educational sports psychology practitioners teach athletes a variety of psychological skills, such as emotional self-control skills with specific concern for arousal regulation and stress-management techniques, attentional control or concentration training, interpersonal skills and abilities that permit them to interact effectively with other athletes and coaches, and goal-setting programs in which athletes learn to appraise and interpret their successes and failures more adequately and effectively.[3] The ultimate goal is to teach athletes how to prepare themselves for competition or endeavor without becoming too anxious or too relaxed; how to monitor their own thoughts, feelings, and images more effectively; and, most important, how to take responsibility for their own actions.

As Terry Orlick points out:

> Sport is a medium which can provide a sense of purpose, a sense of continuous challenge, as well as a range of emotion which is sometimes difficult to experience elsewhere. It can be a rich and meaningful encounter, especially if entered on our own terms. There are few occasions where we have such close contact with other people, with our physical environment, and with ourselves as in sport. There are numerous opportunities for personal growth and for stretching for the limits of human potential, both physically and psychologically.[4]

However, high levels of achievement and excellence in any area do not come easily. There are numerous obstacles to overcome and barriers to push forth. This is particularly true with regard to the injured athlete. Great barriers must be overcome, particularly psychological barriers secondary to the emotional trauma and anxiety associated with the perceived severity of the injury. These may include irrational thoughts and beliefs; attacks on self-image and self-esteem; feelings of helplessness, anger, and depression; and uncertainty surrounding the future.[5]

The purpose of this chapter is to provide the sports medicine practitioner with information and guidelines pertaining to the psychosocial adjustments an athlete might confront following an athletic injury and to provide relevant tools for working more effectively with athletes in the rehabilitation process. The focus of the chapter is on understanding what motivates an athlete to participate in sports; communicating with athletes; the psychological considerations with regard to the injured athlete; and intervention strategies to enhance a sense of psychosocial well-being. Several resources provide a more comprehensive, broader base of knowledge with regard to sport psychology.[1,4,6-14]

UNDERSTANDING MOTIVATION

Motivation is a complex topic in which everyone seems interested and in which many wish to be more knowledgeable. If a room full of coaches is asked how they motivate their athletes, each probably will have a different response.

Some emulate a favorite coach who they read about in the press or watch on television, while others motivate in the way former coaches motivated them. Obviously, numerous techniques and strategies are available from which to choose. Yet motivating an athlete requires far more than just yelling or constantly bombarding him or her with praise or compliments. It requires knowing what are the most important factors influencing the motivational process and how to put this knowledge to its best use.

Perhaps the reason it is so difficult to get a grasp of the subject is that motivation respresents a hypothetical construct not directly observable or measureable, but whose presence can be inferred only indirectly from behavior. Motivation may be thought of as a drive within an individual that serves to arouse, direct, and energize a person's goal-directed behavior.[12,15] Contemporary theories of motivation conceptualize the construct as an interactional process whereupon an individual's behavior is viewed as the result of a continuous interaction between the person and the situation in which he or she finds himself or herself.[1,13,15-17] As Alderman points out, athletes are motivated by factors that lie within them as well as the situation itself.[18] Athletes bring with them unique and different personality characteristics, needs, values, motives, attitudes, expectancies, and abilities to sports situations; these differentially interact with various features of the situation itself, such as practice facilities, task difficulty, level of competition, novelty or change in routine, personality of the coach or trainer, social support from the coach or trainer, or the team's win–loss record. This potential for a variety of interactions can produce different kinds of behavior that will be a direct influence on how motivated that athlete is. Consequently, when it comes to motivating an athlete, coaches and sport medicine practitioners should remember the axiom, "Different strokes for different folks." People and situations differ, so motivational strategies and techniques should be tailored to meet the specific needs of the coach, trainer, and athlete.

To help athletes cope effectively during the process of rehabilitation, it is important to know what goals they have set for themselves and why they continue to participate in sports. What makes all the sacrifices, hard work, and long hours or practice worthwhile? Recently, a number of investigators have begun to identify and examine the major motives, incentives, and reasons why athletes participate in competitive sports. For instance, numerous studies have been conducted on participation motives of young athletes. In general, the research indicates that young athletes have diverse motives for participating in sports, opposed to just one.[15,19-21] These motives include skill development, pursuit of excellence (doing something very well), having fun and seeking excitement, affiliation tendencies (making friends), independence (doing things without the help of others), fitness, power (controlling others), aggression (intimidating others), and success (prestige, status, and recognition). Although the studies cited above dealt with young athletes, the implications for older athletes are apparent. Conversely, Alderman and Wood[19] tested thousands of participants of different ages, sexes, sports, and cultures. From the various motives identified for participation, those consistently rated as most important were pursuit of excellence, skill development, affiliation, excitement, and success.

In regard to group involvement, the literature indicates that individuals join groups because they feel it will satisfy some need or objective that they deem important.[22,23] Common needs include the need for affiliation (friendship, companionship, belongingness), esteem (pride, competence, personal worth), and achievement (recognition, approval, identity). When a group fulfills the needs of its members, individuals often consider the group desirable and membership in that group very valuable. The need for affiliation is often neglected by coaches.[21] Many athletes participate in competitive sport, whether an individual or team sport, because they feel it affords them an opportunity to establish or maintain close personal relationships with people while simultaneously providing them an opportunity to do something well. Thus a coach should create an atmosphere that satisfies an athlete's needs for both excellence and affiliation. In addition to encouraging mastering the fundamentals for athletic excellence, a coach should provide opportunities for an athlete to socialize with teammates so they can develop interpersonal skills essential for the growth and development of psychological well-being.

Hence coaches and trainers must understand their athletes' motives for participating in sports. This understanding comes from careful observation, frequent discussions, recognition of individual differences among athletes, and the development of open lines of communication.[20] It appears that the most important factors that influence sports enjoyment and participation are improvement of skills, being with friends, having fun, a sense of personal accomplishment, and excitement derived from the activity. These findings underscore the fact that the satisfactions and benefits derived from sport are largely intrinsic in nature.

DEVELOPING SELF-MOTIVATION

Intrinsic motivation is behavior motivated by a person's innate need to feel competent and self-determining in dealing with one's surroundings.[24,25] Athletes are intrinsically motivated when they participate for the pure fun, excitement, enjoyment, and pleasure that they derive from the activity itself. Extrinsic motivation implies that performance or participation is controlled by some external force, such as money, awards, trophies, or the coach; if these forces were not present, the individual would cease to engage in that activity or would engage at a reduced rate of quality.[13,26-28]

White[24] proposed that humans are active organisms who seek out challenges from within their environmental surroundings and who strive to be effective in those interactions. He asserts that individuals gain a great deal of satisfaction when they conquer a challenge from within the environment. It is these mastery experiences and subsequent feelings of competence that provide individuals their major source of intrinsic or self-motivation.[29,30] Consequently, the more people feel that their actions reflect a high degree of self-determination and personal competence and that their behavior is caused by their own motives and goals, the higher will be their level of intrinsic motivation. Conversely, if people feel that they are being manipulated or pushed around by others and perceive external incentives to be responsible for controlling their actions, then their intrinsic motivation will be lower.

Hence any efforts to increase a person's intrinsic motivation should be directed toward providing that individual with both a sense of control over his or her own behavior and a feeling of personal accomplishment. An athlete's sense of competence and level of intrinsic motivation can be enhanced through the implementation of goal-setting techniques.[13,22,31-34] Goals affect performance by directing attention and energy to the task at hand, by increasing persistence and continued effort over prolonged periods of time, and by establishing task-relevant strategies for goal attainment. In addition, goals are important because they provide self-evaluative standards from which to judge one's capabilities.[32,33] When people aim for and reach desired levels of performance, they experience a sense of self-satisfaction from knowing they lived up to their own standards of reference.

Certain properties inherent in goals help to provide clear standards of adequacy from which to evaluate progress. Research indicates that goals should be challenging, yet realistic and attainable.[31] Furthermore, goals have been found to be most effective when stated in specific and measurable terms as opposed to vague intentions.[13] A series of short-term proximal goals relating to long-term distal goals should be established with specific target dates for achievement. Whereas long-range goals provide incentive, direction, and evaluation of progress, the attainment of short-term goals provides the athlete with a growing intrinsic sense of pride, personal accomplishment, and self-satisfaction. Since goals are dynamic in nature,[13] periodic evaluations should be undertaken to ensure that the goals that have been set are difficult enough to challenge yet realistic enough to achieve. Worthwhile outcomes come from hard work and planning. Goals provide us with standards to do our best, to find out what we are and are not capable of achieving.

The discussion thus far has focused on teaching individuals the importance of taking responsibility for their own actions in their quest for athletic excellence. In essence, personal excellence is a by-product of believing in one's capabilities and performing with a sense of pride, commitment, tenacity, and determination to reach identified goals and objectives.[4,22] However, a belief in one's capabilities is only as good as its execution. A factor that appears to be crucial in achieving personal excellence is an individual's level of self-efficacy or self-confidence. Self-efficacy is defined as the strength of one's conviction that he or she can successfully execute a behavior required to produce a certain outcome.[33] Efficacy expectations determine how much effort people expend on a task and how long they will persist in the face of adversity or setbacks. Assuming that an individual is capable of a response and that appropriate incentives are available for optimal performance, efficacy theory asserts than an individual's actual performance will be predicted by his or her feeling of competence or expectation or personal effectiveness. Consequently, if athletes can set a series of specific, measurable, yet attainable goals that are just far enough ahead to require continuous improvement and effort, then the corresponding success will build confidence in their capabilities. Additionally, research from attribution theory reinforces the same point: if success in sport is perceived to be the result of internal personal factors, such as ability, effort, and training hard, then emotional feelings of pride, satisfaction, effectiveness, and competence derived from attaining previously set goals provide an important vehicle for the development of perceived levels of efficacy.[35–41] Thus if the idea is to enhance within the athlete a sense of pride and responsibility (for his or her actions), then goal-setting techniques and positive expectancies represent an excellent vehicle for enhancement of intrinsic motivation and feelings of efficacy and control over adverse situations.

ENHANCING MOTIVATION THROUGH COMMUNICATION

The physical therapist and athletic trainer deal with motivation by getting to know each athlete as a unique individual so that, if injured, they can instill within the athlete desirable attitudes and patterns of response toward rehabilitation training that promote positive reconditioning. If the goal or rehabilitation is to get the athlete back to the playing field quickly and safely, then learning how to communicate effectively and establishing a desirable rapport with athletes becomes an area of vital concern to the sports medicine practitioner.

Communication is a two-way venture, so both the athlete and sports medicine practitioner have a joint responsibility to make it work. The foundation for effective communication is trust, credibility, and mutual respect.[22] Credibility is reflected in the athlete's attitude about the trustworthiness of what you say and the manner in which the message is conveyed. For instance, the content of a message (i.e., what is actually said) is not always as important as how it is said (i.e., the voice intonations and nonverbal mannerisms associated with the way the message is expressed emotionally). Similarly, one of the most important skills one can learn to develop is communicating in a positive manner. The positive approach emphasizes praise and rewards to strengthen desirable behaviors as opposed to the negative approach, which uses fear, punishment, and criticism to eliminate undesirable behaviors. According to Martens et al.,[10] the positive approach is "an attitude that communicates a desire to understand, an acceptance of others, and an expectation of mutual respect." This can be accomplished by being reliable, fair, nonjudgmental, and consistent, by showing the athlete a genuine concern about their overall welfare, and by making every member of the team feel valued, important, and special. Hence the positive approach helps athletes feel good about themselves as individuals, which in turn gives the sports medicine practitioner credibility in their eyes.[10,42]

Communication consists of both sending and receiving verbal and nonverbal messages. In fact, it has been estimated that more than 70 percent of our actions are communicated nonverbally in the form of gestures, body move-ments, spatial relationships, and facial expressions. In general, most people seem to be quite proficient at talking and sending messages. However, the area of communication that usually needs the most work is the art of listening and striving to understand what is really being said.[9,10] The key to developing good listening skills is to be an active, responsive listener.[10,42] This can be accomplished by showing the athlete concern; by making good eye contact when communicating; by giving undivided attention; by probing judiciously to facilitate problem clarification and self-exploration skills; by responding with respect and empathy to what the athlete has to say; and by developing a good rapport with the athletes.[42]

Establishing a good rapport with athletes is an important interpersonal skill and area of communication that needs to be developed.[43,44] Rapport can be nurtured by establishing open lines of communication that reflect trust, mutual respect, concern, and encouragement. This in turn should build confidence in the athletes' mind that the sports medicine practitioner is a good and competent person. In addition, a good rapport sets the stage for the healthy exchange of ideas and emotions relevant to the injury itself.

The goals of the rehabilitation process actually can be hampered by the emotional state and beliefs of the injured athlete. Emotions such as fear, anxiety, anger, frustration, and disappointment are normal reactions to a traumatic injury. The first step is to make certain the athlete understands exactly the nature of the injury. The diagnosis and problem should be explained in language the athlete can comprehend easily. Athletes should be allowed the opportunity to express their anxieties and concerns and to ask any questions they may have in an empathetic atmosphere so they are not left wondering or uncertain about what to expect. Accurate and honest information, padded with verbal and non-verbal expressions of hope, should help the athlete deal with their emotional feelings more effectively.

Once rapport is established and diagnosis completed, the next step is to develop a positive attitude within the athlete that is conducive to the goals that are important for proper rehabilitation (i.e., to gain a range of motion, strength, power, flexibility, muscular endurance, cardiovascular endurance, speed, balance, agility, and skill). Recovery is usually a rather slow and often tedious process. Although many injured athletes lack patience, their interest in recovery must be aroused. They must be made aware both of what needs to be done to correct their problem and that results will be determined largely by the energy and enthusiasm they put into the reconditioning program.

The process associated with rehabilitation comprises many steps, and each one must be completed successfully and without pain before the athlete can return to competition. Criteria for return are established for each injury in terms of skills and abilities the athlete will need to regain before returning to his or her sport. The athlete must be told what these criteria are so that he or she can have concrete goals toward which to strive. Thus it is suggested that the sports medicine practitioner provide athletes with a blueprint or game plan to work from so they have a clear, realistic idea of what to expect at each stage of the rehabilitation program. Furthermore, the rehabilitation program should be broken down into small, manageable units so the athlete can have short-term, attainable daily and weekly goals to achieve along the way.

Once the rehabilitation program is clearly delineated, the sports medicine practitioner should establish a realistic time frame for recovery. Since each athlete differs in terms of belief systems and the amount of pain he or she can tolerate, one should avoid giving a specific time period for healing. The goal is to return the athlete to the same activity level as before the injury occurred in the shortest amount of time possible. It will take a commitment and positive attitude on the part of the athlete, along with patience, persistent effort, and will power to want to succeed to make the recovery work.

Thus the ability to communicate effectively with each athlete, to relate to the athletes' needs and concerns, and to identify and empathize with the struggles and pressures that the injury and corresponding sense of inactivity place on the athlete are all important factors in striving to develop a desirable attitude within the athlete of wanting to get better.

COPING WITH INJURY

Injuries have both physical and psychological effects on an athlete. Although numerous articles have been written on the physical aspect of athletic injuries and the subsequent stages of rehabilitation, a dearth of literature exists concerning the psychological side of athletic injuries. An exception is an excellent article written by Robert Rotella,[5] who pointed out that typical psychological reactions to an injury quite often progress through states similar to those of a person coping with the loss of a loved one. Initially, athletes might respond to an injury with a sense of denial and disbelief, thinking that nothing's wrong with them and that the injury will get better after a good night's rest. As they become more aware of the extent of their injury, they advance through stages of anger, frustration, bargaining, depression, grief, and finally acceptance and abdication that the injury does exist. Yet they still must remain positive, enthusiastic, and hopeful about the prospect for total recovery.[5]

For instance, following the stage of disbelief, it is common for athletes to respond to an injury with anger, blame, and self-condemnation, becoming irritated not only with themselves but with others as well. A baseball catcher who learns that he suffered a dislocated shoulder trying to prevent a runner from scoring may blame himself for not blocking the plate properly, the outfielder for not getting the ball to him quickly enough, or the opponent for a "dirty" hit. Soon, frustration sets in when the athlete realizes that the injury represents the difference between actively competing and passively watching as a spectator on the sidelines. Bargaining follows with the rationalization that "yes, I am injured, but I better be able to compete again come playoff time." The true sense of loss and despair may cause athletes to become depressed, as evidenced by retreating within themselves, wallowing in self-pity, feeling sorry for themselves, and perhaps becoming anxious or guilt-ridden that they can't contribute to the productivity of the team. Following this "period of mourning" comes the time for the athlete to move on, learning how to put things in proper perspective and accept the injury for what it is. The focus should be on keeping expectations flexible and goals realistic. The athlete should be taught to respond like a true champion, with a sense of pride, confidence, and renewed determination. Consequently, the goal of the athletic trainer or physical therapist is to shorten the amount of time that it takes the athlete to move from the initial stage of disbelief to that of acceptance.[5]

Individual differences exist among athletes with regard to the way they perceive injuries and cope with pain. For instance, Rotella noted that although one athlete may perceive an injury as disastrous, another may perceive it as an opportunity to display self-discipline, persistence, and courage to fight back.[5] Along these lines, a variety of situational factors can interact with personality characteristics of athletes to influence the way they cope with injuries. For some athletes, the agony associated with watching their teammates dress for a big game or the feeling of helplessness associated with the loss of opportunity to display their athletic skills often serves as an impetus that ignites their inner drive to rehabilitate themselves properly and get back to the playing field quickly. Conversely, athletes who are looking for an easy way out may perceive an injury as solace from the embarrassment of unsatisfactory performance or from the frustration associated with going through a losing season. Hence the emphasis again is on developing appropriate communication skills, striving to "reach the chord" within each individual to find out and understand what makes him or her tick. Time spent getting to know athletes is time well spent: respect is earned, anxiety concerning the athletes' emotional response to injury is reduced, and cooperation and trust is gained.

PSYCHOLOGICAL INTERVENTION STRATEGIES

In recent years, there has been a rapid growth in the application of self-control strategies to enhance sport performance.[2,8,45–47] This is not surprising, since in the stress-filled world of sports athletes are often required simultaneously to cope with great pressures, adapt to a variety of changing conditions, and maintain poise, discipline, and concentration under trying circumstances. With any injury, numerous physical, psychological, and emotional obstacles must be overcome on the road to recovery. The final section of this chapter highlights various stress-management and psychological intervention strategies that can be used to help the athlete cope more effectively with injury. One or all of these strategies may be used in work with athletes.

Emotional Self-control

Perhaps the single most important coping skill athletes can have at their disposal is emotional self-control.[5] From a sports psychologist's perspective, emotional self-control deals with teaching athletes how to manage stress, anxiety, and arousal more effectively in their pursuit of athletic excellence. Stress is a subjectively defined event that involves an interaction among cognitive, somatic, and behavioral systems, often elicited by perceived emotional or physical threat.[48] Cognitively, stress or anxiety manifests itself in terms of a narrowing of the perceptual field (i.e., inappropriate focus of attention) and a preoccupation with irrational emotional thoughts that usually reflect fear, apprehension, worry, and self-doubt. When we worry, we tend to focus on the undesireable aspects of a situation and the negative consequences that might result. Physiologically, stress manifests itself in terms of increased activation of the autonomic nervous system, evidenced by increased heart rate and respiratory rate, nervousness, and muscle tension. Learning to manage one's emotional reaction to stress is a psychophysiological skill that takes practice to be perfected.[2,3] The sports medicine practitioner can teach an athlete more effectively to manage stress and his or her reaction to it by: (1) helping athletes examine and understand the specific things that cause them to be stressed; (2) helping athletes break down their stress response into a series of component phases that they can learn to control; and (3) providing athletes with the needed coping skills that will enable them to regulate their thoughts, feelings, and attitudes more appropriately from a self-enhancing, as opposed to self-defeating, perspective.

For example, it is not unusual for an athlete to become overwhelmed by anxiety-induced emotions and maladaptive thought patterns when a severe injury occurs. Football players who experience an anterior cruciate ligament tear 2 days before the big game may initially perceive the situation as catastrophic, convincing themselves that they have let down the coach and teammates, that their season is over, and that they will never be able to perform effectively again. Rather than viewing the situation as hopeless and being overwhelmed by the potential consequences associated with the perceived severity of the injury, athletes with emotional self-control can cope with the ACL tear in a rational, self-enhancing manner, first by acknowledging the specific things that are causing them to be stressed (hurt, frustration, disappointment that the injury came at an unfortunate and inconvenient time), but then by reinterpreting the setback in a more adequate and constructive way so they remain positive, in control, and determined to get better. The coping skills the athlete may incorporate to take control over the situation may include relaxation and deep-breathing exercises to reduce physiological activation levels, attitude restructuring techniques to help increase awareness of inner speech and to become psychologically sensitive to faulty dialogue, and a goal-setting program to provide motivation and direction and a vehicle from which to succeed and experience a sense of personal accomplishment.

Athletes with emotional self-control view injury as a temporary setback. Rather than be overwhelmed by the severity of the injury, they respond to it in an emotionally mature, rational manner. They realize that rehabilitation will be long and demanding, challenging both their self-discipline and will power. But if they have the desire and commitment to be the best athlete they can be and want to reach the goals that they have outlined for themselves, then they can't let the injury stand in their way. They must have confidence in their ability to overcome this challenge. They must develop a positive belief that with pride, determination, and hard work (i.e., the same psychological qualities that helped them excel on the athletic field), they will come back from injury a better athlete than they were before.

One final note on emotional self-control. Rehabilitation can often be a very long and demanding process. Hence it is not unusual for an athlete to vacillate through emotional highs and lows, appearing to be up one day, down the next. Furthermore, they may go through plateau periods when they don't see improvement for weeks. The sports medicine practitioner can help athletes during these down times by directing their attention toward the intrinsic reasons and emotional highs they derive from sport participation in the first place: the joy, excitement, and aesthetic qualities of sport; the pride and satisfaction of personal accomplishment; the excitement and enthusiasm associated with doing something well; the tremendous friendships and camaraderie that sport offers. Likewise, if athletes are having trouble with their "attitude muscle" and level of motivation during plateau periods, a sports medicine practitioner can do a variety of things to help the athlete regain a sense of emotional self-control:

1. Be sure that the athlete has realistic expectations. It is unrealistic for an athlete to think that he or she should see daily improvement in a linear fashion, because some days will be better than others.

2. Help the athlete redefine goals that are consistent with the current level of improvement. Injured athletes often want to know how long they will be out of action or when they can return to competition. This question can create much stress. A goal-setting program that focuses on short-term goals in relation to long-term objectives will give athletes something tangible to aim toward and will leave them with a sense of accomplishment and personal control over the situation.

3. Teach athletes to accept responsibility for their own actions. Successful rehabilitation takes pride, patience, persistence, and hard work. Successful athletes not only think they will get better, they believe they will get better. Accordingly, they strive to make the most out of each and every situation, rhetorically asking themselves: "What did I do today to help myself improve and become a better athlete?"

4. Try to communicate in a positive manner. Reward, encourage, and praise injured athletes frequently and sincerely throughout the rehabilitation program. In addition, reward the little things along the way. Make them feel good about the way they define their own self-concepts.[43]

5. Encourage athletes to look to others for emotional support. When faced with a serious injury, support and encouragement from family, friends, team members, and sports medicine personnel can give athletes the strength to overcome difficult obstacles.[5] Injured athletes also can gain inspiration and support from others by reading books or case studies of other injured athletes who have overcome great odds and returned to competition.

Relaxation Training

An extremely important self-control skill for the injured athlete is the ability to relax. Two things happen during most relaxation procedures. Physiologically, muscles become less tense; heart rate slows down; and blood pressure, respiratory rate, and oxygen consumption decrease.[49] Psychologically, relaxation promotes positive feelings of calm, creativity, concentration, confidence, and self-control. The injured athlete may use relaxation training as a tool to control pain, alleviate anxiety, combat stress, temper anger, or enhance his or her self-image.

Progressive Relaxation. One of the more popular techniques sports psychologists use to teach athletes how to relax is Jacobson's Progressive Relaxation Training Exercise.[50] Progressive relaxation training is a systematic method of teaching comprehensive skeletal muscle relaxation and is designed to help the athlete recognize and get rid of unnecessary muscular tension in the body. In essence, athletes are taught alternately to contract, then relax major muscle groups in the body in a systematic and orderly sequence (i.e., hands, biceps and triceps, shoulders, neck, facial area, chest, stomach, buttocks, thighs, calves, feet, and toes). They become able to differentiate how their muscles feel when they are tense or relaxed, thereby sensitizing them to proprioceptive feedback from these muscles. The goal of training is to help athletes become more aware of personal signs of tension and know how to release the unwanted tension when necessary. Although there are many variations, Orlick[4] and Wolpe and Lazarus[51] give excellent instructions for the implementation of Jacobson's technique.

Deep-breathing Exercise. Deep-breathing exercises also have been noted to be an important part of relaxation training.[9,52] Breathing is important because many athletes don't know how to breathe properly. Often when an athlete is asked by the coach to relax and take a deep breath, the response is incorrect, as evidenced by inefficient, forceful breathing from the shoulders and chest as opposed to slow, steady breathing from the diaphragm. With deep diaphragmatic and lower costal breathing, each breath originates from the diaphragm and moves its way up toward the chest in a slow, steady progression.[52] The abdomen should rise with inhalation and recede with exhalation. Initially, it is good for the athlete to rest the hands on the stomach so he or she can feel the abdomen move properly. Inhalation should be slow, steady, and deep through the nostrils until the diaphragm and lungs fill completely with air. Exhalation should be through the mouth, following the same procedure in reverse order. Attention should be focused on the smooth transition of rhythmical breathing, increasing the sensation of relaxation with each inhalation, and releasing as much tension as possible with each exhalation. The result of this type of breathing is a calm, soothing effect that leaves the individual relaxed and centered.

Cue-controlled Relaxation. Deep diaphragmatic breathing exercises coupled with cue-controlled self-instructional statements are an excellent way to strengthen one's relaxation response.[4,8,9,51,53] For instance, in cue-controlled relaxation, athletes are taught to repeat the word "calm," "relax," "stay cool," or anything else that holds appropriate meaning to them each time they exhale. At the end of modified progressive relaxation programs, athletes should be instructed to repeat whatever word works well for them 20 to 30 times in a row, trying to relax more fully each time they say it. The goal is to try to strengthen the association between the cue word and total relaxation so that when the athlete is confronted with stress during the heat of competition, he or she can use the cue word to start the relaxation process.

Perhaps an example will clarify the picture. A basketball player is fouled with 2 seconds remaining in the game; the team is down by one point. Rather than get upset by the criticality of the situation, the athlete incorporates a cue-controlled relaxation response to help reduce the anxiety to a manageable level. Before approaching the foul line, the athlete takes two deep, relaxing breaths from the diaphragm, repeating the cue word "RE-LAX" slowly during each exhalation. Quickly, the athlete scans the body for any excess signs of tension, uses the centered breathing technique to flow relaxation to that spot, steps up to the line confident and relaxed, and proceeds to hit both free throws to win the game.

The goal of cue-controlled relaxation is to teach the athlete how to achieve a state of relaxation in response to a self-produced cue word. Cues also can be used to enhance or maintain performance; for example, an alpine skier may think "attack the course" prior to performance.[8,54] Either way, the key to cue-instructional responses is associating the desired response with its appropriate cue.

Other Relaxation Techniques.   Many other methods have been found to be quite beneficial in helping an athlete to learn to relax. Autogenic training,[55] biofeedback,[56,57] and meditation[58] are just a few techniques that may be appropriate in given situations, but they often require greater motivation and self-discipline to be effective.

Autogenic training was originally developed in Germany in the 1920s by Schultz and Luthe[55] and has been quite popular in Europe. In its basic form, autogenic training consists of six standard exercises composed of a combination of relaxation and self-suggestion techniques. The first exercise is devoted to the cultivation of sensations of heaviness in the limbs (muscular relaxation), the second to sensations of warmth (peripheral dilation), the third to reduction of heart rate, the fourth to development of a smooth regular pattern of respiration, the fifth to visceral regulation with emphasis on cultivating warmth in the solar plexus, and the sixth to cooling the forehead. This series of exercises is designed to produce deep relaxation and restore homeostasis in the body.

A technique that has become popular in recent years is *biofeedback*.[56,57] Through instrumentation, the athlete receives physiological feedback (e.g., peripheral skin temperature, muscle tension, and blood pressure) that indicates his or her present state of tension. By trial and error with feedback reinforcement, the athlete learns to control these variables for optimal functioning. At first, instrumentation helps the athlete recognize when he or she is tense, observe the cause of tension, and develop techniques to reduce the tension. Once the skill has been mastered, the athlete should be able to induce the desired state of relaxation at will without the use of the instrument. Although bio-feedback training has been found to be an effective tool from which to enhance the learning of self-regulation skills, most coaches and trainers do not have the equipment available to them or the expertise to use it properly.

Regardless of which technique is chosen, the important point is that re-laxation is a skill. As such, practice is essential to gain competence.

Imagery Training

An excellent self-control strategy many athletes use to reduce anxiety or enhance concentration is imagery, or mental rehearsal training.[4,8,59] Many world-class athletes have reported that they try mentally to picture themselves going through their actual movements in their minds just prior to performance. For example, world diving champion and Olympic gold medalist Greg Louganis is a master at imagery training. He visualizes his dives perfectly, rehearses them to music, and coordinates his timing with auditory recall. Jack Nicklaus has often said that he never hits a golf ball without first visualizing himself hitting the ball. Dwight Stones and Dick Fosbury, before they high-jump, see and feel themselves accelerating toward the bar, planting their foot, then clear-ing the bar successfully. I could present numerous other anecdotes, but the point is that many top athletes psychologically and emotionally program their muscles for peak performance. Imagery techniques also are a powerful tool to help athletes cope effectively while recovering from an injury.

Imagery is a "covert activity whereby a person experiences sensory-motor sensations that reintegrate reality experiences."[59] Imagery serves as a mental blueprint to enhance one's perceptual experience. It is an appropriate technique to help athletes set goals for themselves, control emotions, develop self-aware-ness, relieve pain, or practice sports skills. For some athletes, imagery serves as a last-minute reminder of the pattern they wish to reproduce. For others, it takes their minds off any negative thoughts of worry or self-doubt, reaffirming a last-second feeling of confidence prior to performance.

Typically, visualization exercises are facilitated by the use of relaxation training. Relaxation allows athletes the opportunity to develop more vivid and productive visual images.

Imagery is more than just visual. It is a polysensory modality, involving the tactile, auditory, visual, emotional, and muscular systems. Thus, when imaging, an athlete should try to recreate the desired experience with as much sensual feeling as possible (e.g., see the playing arena, feel the sweat, smell the gym, hear the crowd, feel himself or herself developing a kinesthetic mus-cular response as he or she experiences the feelings associated with the move-ment itself). The more specific and detailed the image, the better will be its effect.

Unfortunately, there is not enough space in this chapter to explore fully the mechanics of imagery training. Richard Suinn has developed a relaxation–imagery package, visual–motor behavioral rehearsal (VMBR), that is a popular intervention technique used in sports to help athletes manage stress and improve concentration.[8] Numerous books and articles are designed to teach an individual how to image properly.[4,8,59-61]

Imagery also can be used as a coping tool during injury rehabilitation. First, it can be used to keep the athlete mentally fresh and alert while recovering from an injury. For instance, a wide receiver sidelined for 2 to 3 weeks with a severe ankle sprain can keep himself mentally alert by vividly going over plays in his mind. A typical scenario might go something like this: The wide receiver could hear the play called in the huddle; feel confident and self-assured as he approaches the line of scrimmage; tune into the kinesthetic feel of running a crisp pass pattern, catching the ball, getting hit by the cornerback, then bouncing up off the ground feeling great about the way the play was executed. The process starts over again with each new play. Similarly, electromyographic research indicates that although the athlete is not physically practicing the skill in question, neurological impulses and small contractions can be measured in the muscles associated with the movements being imaged.[4] Thus when an individual imagines something vividly, his or her body responds as if it were real. Consequently, imagery can enhance neuromuscular functioning even in the absence of physical practice.

Earlier, I suggested that the sports medicine practitioner provide the athlete with a blueprint or game plan to work from so the athlete understands exactly the nature of the injury and has a clear, realistic idea of what to expect at each stage of the rehabilitation program. Furthermore, I suggested that the rehabilitation program be broken down into small, manageable units so the athlete could have short-term attainable goals to aim for along the way. Imagery training could be used to help athletes "see the big picture" in terms of the nature of their injury, what must occur inside their body if healing is to take place, and the steps involved in the rehabilitation program. The athletes can then use imagery techniques to visualize healing taking place inside the body and develop appropriate daily and weekly goals whereupon they can see themselves completing sequential steps in the rehabilitation process on their road to recovery.[62] Consequently, they will have a cognitive understanding of what is going on inside their body during convalescence and have something productive to look forward to in terms of specific, outlined rehabilitation goals to be accomplished.

Imagery can be used as a pain-control strategy as well. If the athlete is experiencing a great deal of pain while being treated for an injury, the person can disassociate himself or herself from the situation, and in his or her own mind be somewhere pleasant, satisfying, and enjoyable, such as walking along the beach at sunset or sitting next to a waterfall in the mountains.

Finally, imagery training can be used to develop positive attitudes in emotionally drained athletes. In this situation, motivation can be enhanced by having the injured athlete rekindle images and emotions associated with past successes in sports.

Imagery techniques can be used by an injured athlete to practice sports skills mentally, to develop self-awareness, to remain positively oriented, and to reduce anxiety and enhance concentration. Furthermore, it provides a motivational framework from which to develop positive attitudes and expectancies that are very important to the rehabilitation process. "In your mind, you can learn to see yourself, hear yourself, feel yourself, and think yourself through potentially stressful situations in a positive, constructive manner."[4]

Systematic Desensitization

Occasionally following a severe injury, an athlete will require more counseling and assistance in preparation for a safe and successful recovery. Athletes exhibiting definite performance decrements following an accident (getting hit in the head with a 95-mph baseball) or injury (hitting the head on a high diving board) may need to overcome their fears, anxieties, and other psychological scars associated with the previously painful experience.[5,63] When conditioned emotionality interferes with performance, counterconditioning techniques should be used.[45] Systematic desensitization represents a counterconditioning, self-control strategy designed to help individuals effectively handle a particular fear or anxiety. It appears to be a viable technique for psychologically and emotionally rehabilitating the injured athlete.[64,65] According to Wolpe, anxious people have learned through a process of classical conditioning to experience excessively high levels of sympathetic nervous system arousal in the presence of certain stimuli. The goal of treatment is to replace sympathetic activity with competing behaviors that have a predominance of parasympathetic innervation, a process called reciprocal inhibition.[64] In systematic desensitization, relaxation is used as the incompatible response to permit the gradual counterconditioning of fear and anxiety.[63]

Desensitization requires a careful assessment of the situations that elicit fear and anxiety. First, the athlete is trained to achieve a deep, physiological state of relaxation. At the same time relaxation is being mastered, the athlete and practitioner/coach begin to construct a graded hierarchy of 10 to 15 anxiety-provoking situations, arranged in ascending order in terms of the intensity of anxiety they elicit (from little or no anxiety to extremely threatening). For instance, the following represents a shortened graded fear hierarchy for a football running back returning to action toward the end of the season after missing 4 weeks due to a severe knee sprain.

1. The trainer informs you that you are ready to return to competition.
2. You return to practice scrimmaging without pads.
3. In the middle of the week, you being practicing with pads in a situation where you are actually getting tackled by teammates.
4. You are getting taped in the training room, 2 hours before the game.
5. You are warming up on the field, practicing wind sprints and cutbacks.
6. You receive handoffs while practicing off-tackle plays with your offensive unit.

7. You are standing on the sideline prior to kickoff.
8. You are in the huddle and have been asked to block for the other running back on the first play from scrimmage.
9. You are in the huddle on the next play and have been asked to carry the ball on a misdirection play.
10. Midway through the second quarter, you break away on a sweep and the free safety catches you from behind, tackling you directly on the knee.

When the athlete has mastered the relaxation skill and the hierarchy has been developed, treatment begins. The athlete's task is to maintain the relaxed state while simultaneously concentrating on the visualized image or scene. The athlete begins with stimuli that generate the least amount of anxiety and gradually progresses to visualizing situations that result in increasing amounts of anxiety. If any noticeable signs of tension or anxiety are felt, the athlete raises his or her hand and concentrates once again on the relaxation exercise. The pairing of the situation with relaxation continues until each situation in order has been overcome successfully. The criterion for progression to situations arousing increased anxiety is the consistent maintenance of a relaxed state in the face of the anxiety-provoking situation at the preceding level of the hierarchy. Systematic desensitization would be most effective if used in conjunction with electromyographic biofeedback equipment as an extremely sensitive and objective measure of muscle tension and relaxation. Wolpe and Lazarus[51] provide a comprehensive review of systematic desensitization.

Cognitive Behavioral Intervention Packages

The skills involved in coping with injury and illness are many and varied.[5,6] People and situations are different, so response to treatment varies based on the interaction between the two. Hence the most successful implementation of an intervention program requires flexibility and diversity on the part of the sports medicine practitioner. A variety of self-control intervention programs that will help an athlete assume more personal responsibility for his or her own actions and cope more effectively with stress, anxiety, injury, or illness is available.[66] Following is a brief description of various cognitive–behavioral intervention programs that have been used successfully with athletes. The original references provide more detailed descriptions.

Cognitive Restructuring and Rational Thinking. Cognitive restructuring is a coping skill strategy designed to help athletes become more attuned to their own thinking patterns in times of stress. Athletes often react to the stress of being injured in an emotional, irrational manner. According to Smith: "a powerful means of reducing maladaptive emotional responses from anxiety-induced situations is to modify the cognitions that elicit and reinforce emotionality."[45] Perhaps the best approaches to changing maladaptive thought patterns are Ellis' rational emotive therapy,[67] Meichenbaum's stress inoculation training,[68] and Smith's cognitive–affective stress management training.[69]

In rational emotive therapy, Ellis proposes that the relationship among thoughts, emotions, and behaviors follows an A–B–C paradigm: A represents a situation or experience; B, the assumptions an individual makes about that experience; C, the feelings and behaviors that result not from the experience itself but rather from the assumptions about the experience. For example, if a shortstop dislocates a shoulder sliding into second base right before the playoffs and feels terrible about it, he or she might assume that dislocating the shoulder caused the terrible feelings. Ellis would argue that it was not the injury but the assumptions about the consequences associated with the injury that caused the terrible feelings (i.e., not being able to contribute to the productivity of the team come playoff time, letting teammates down). At point D, an examination and dispute of the irrational assumptions made at point B would be made, allowing a substitution of a more rational thought at point E.

Stress Inoculation Training. Whereas rational emotive therapy teaches individuals to construe external events in a rational adaptive way, stress inoculation training[68] is designed to help an individual develop the cognitive ability to recognize faulty self-statements made prior to and during stressful situations. Through self-instructional training, the person is able to substitute more adaptive positive self-statements when dealing with stressors. As its name implies, stress inoculation training is a comprehensive immunization package that incorporates both cognitive and physiological coping skills that an individual can master to inoculate himself or herself against stress.

The procedure involves three phases. The first phase is an educational phase, designed to provide the individual with an explanation of how stress occurs and his or her reaction to it. The individual is taught to perceive stress as a series of phases rather than as one overwhelming experience (i.e., recognition of heightened physiological arousal followed by maladaptive thoughts such as fear, pain, anger, and being overwhelmed by the stressor).

The second phase is the rehearsal phase, when the therapist/practitioner provides the individual with adaptive coping skills to deal with perceived stressors. The coping skills include physical relaxation, learning ways in which others cope, monitoring self-statements by being taught to replace maladaptive, negative self-statements with adaptive, positive self-statements. Specific sets of self-statements are developed for various phases[70]: (1) preparing for a stressor (the athlete analyzes the situation: "What is it I have to do? Think rationally and believe in the ability I possess."); (2) confronting the stressor ("Relax, you're in control, take a few deep breaths of relaxation, then focus in on what it is I have to do to be successful."); (3) coping with feelings of being overwhelmed at critical moments ("If overaroused, just pause, take a few deep breaths, slow things down, keep focused on what it is I have to do."); and (4) reinforcing self-statements for effective coping ("Great job—I knew I could do it").

The third phase is the application, designed to give the individual an opportunity to practice newly acquired coping skills in a stressful situation. Stressful situations are introduced in a graduated fashion, often proceeding from imaginary to real-life situations. Stress inoculation training has been used successfully to reduce fear, anxiety, and anger, as well as to increase tolerance to pain.[68,71] It would appear to be highly applicable to athletes as well.

Cognitive–Affective Stress Management.   Smith's cognitive–affective stress management training[69] is similar to Meichenbaum's program in that it involves the acquisition and rehearsal of both cognitive coping skills and relaxation skills. The major difference between the two approaches lies in the methods used to rehearse coping skills once they have been acquired. As Smith points out:

> rather than rehearsing under low levels of anxiety as in the inoculation model, a technique known as induced affect is employed to allow rehearsal of coping responses under high emotional arousal. The client is asked to imagine a stressful situation, then focus on the feeling that the scene elicits.[45]

Verbal suggestions that feelings are growing more intense are used to shape a strong affective response.[72] When highly aroused, the individual is taught to incorporate an integrated coping response to control the stress that includes somatic relaxation, rhythmical diaphragmatic breathing exercises, and positive self-statements. As the individual inhales, a task-relevant, stress-reducing self-statement is emitted. On exhalation, the individual is taught to give a mental self-instruction to relax, thus inducing somatic relaxation (similar to cue-controlled relaxation).

Other Self-regulation Models.   Several other multifaceted cognitive–behavioral intervention packages have been shown to promote effective and long-lasting self-regulation skills in athletes. Suinn[8] and Spinelli and Barrios[73] have utilized a technique known as visual motor behavioral rehearsal (VMBR), which emphasizes the use of relaxation and imagery techniques to improve athletic performance. Silva[54] has developed a three-phase cognitive behavioral training program to assist athletes in the modification of the performance problem. In the identification phase, each athlete is asked to identify in detail the specific problem he or she wants modified along with the covert verbalizations and images they experience before, during, and after the behavior is performed. Next, in the cognitive restructuring phase, the process of attitude change is undertaken. In the final phase, the pairing phase, a concentration cue word is paired with a covertly conditioned image to produce desired responses. Kirschenbaum and associates[47,74] developed a five-phase model of self-regulation that appears to be extremely generalizable to sport situations. Two of the more important components of this cognitive behavioral intervention program are positive self-monitoring techniques and positive expectancies about the likelihood of achieving one's goals.

SUMMARY

The focus of this chapter was to provide the sports medicine practitioner with information and guidelines pertaining to the psychological adjustments an athlete might confront following an athletic injury. The emphasis was placed on developing appropriate communication skills and fostering positive expectations that reflect on the part of the athlete the desire to get better. A variety of psychological intervention strategies, such as cue-controlled relaxation, imagery training, attitude restructuring, and goal-setting programs were presented as self-control techniques that can be used to help the athlete cope more effectively with injury.

REFERENCES

1. Silva J, Weinberg R: Psychological Foundations of Sport. Human Kinetics Publishers, Champaign, 1984
2. Waitley D, May J, Martens R: Sport psychology and the elite athlete. p. 87. In Zarius B (ed): Clinics in Sports Medicine. WB Saunders, Philadelphia, 1983
3. Martens R: How sport psychology can help Olympic athletes. Paper presented at the Olympic Symposium, Skidmore College, Saratoga Springs, 1980
4. Orlick T: In Pursuit of Athletic Excellence. Human Kinetics Publishers, Champaign, 1980
5. Rotella R: Psychological care of the injured athlete. p. 213. In Kuland D (ed): The Injured Athlete. JB Lippincott, Philadelphia, 1982
6. Straub W: Sport Psychology: An Analysis of Athlete Behavior. Mouvement Publications, Ithaca, 1978
7. Straub W, Williams J: Cognitive Sport Psychology. Sport Science Associates, Lansing, 1984
8. Suinn R: Psychology in Sports: Methods and Applications. Burgess Publishing, Minneapolis, 1980
9. Harris D, Harris B: The Athlete's Guide to Sports Psychology: Mental Skills for Physical People. Leisure Press, New York, 1984
10. Martens R, Christina R, Harvey J, Sharkey B: Coaching Young Athletes. Human Kinetics Publishers, Champaign, 1981
11. Smoll F, Smith R (eds): Psychological Perspectives in Youth Sports. Hemisphere Publishing, Washington, 1978
12. Carron A: Social Psychology of Sport. Mouvement Publications, Ithaca, 1980
13. Carron A: Motivation: Implications for Coaching and Teaching. Sports Dynamics, London, Canada, 1984
14. Rushall B: Psyching in Sports. Pelham Books, London, 1979
15. Landers D: Motivation and performance: the role of arousal and attentional factors. p. 91. In Straub W (ed): Sport Psychology: An Analysis of Athlete Behavior. Mouvement Publications, Ithaca, 1978
16. Endler N, Magnusson D (eds): Interactional Psychology and Personality. Hemisphere Publishers, Washington, D.C., 1976
17. Bunker L, Rotella R: Achievement and stress in sport: research findings and practical suggestions. p. 104. In Straub W (ed): Sport Psychology: An Analysis of Athlete Behavior. Mouvement Publications, Ithaca, 1978
18. Alderman R: Incentive motivation in sport: an interpretive speculation of research opportunities. p. 146. In Fisher C (ed): Psychology of Sport. Mayfield Publishing, Palo Alto, 1976
19. Alderman R, Wood N: An analysis of incentive motivation in young Canadian athletes. Can J Appl Sport Sci 1:169, 1976

20. Gould D, Horn T: Participation motivation in young athletes. p. 359. In Silva J, Weinberg R (eds): Psychological Foundations of Sport. Human Kinetics Publishers, Champaign, 1984
21. Passer M: Children in sport: participation motives and psychological stress. Quest, 33:231, 1981
22. Yukelson D: Group motivation in sport teams. p. 229. In Silva J, Weinberg R (eds): Psychological Foundations of Sport. Human Kinetics Publishers, Champaign, 1984
23. Shaw M: Group Dynamics: The Psychology of Small Group Behavior. 2nd Ed. McGraw–Hill, New York, 1976
24. White R: Motivation reconsidered: the concept of competence. Psychol Rev, 66:297, 1959
25. Deci E: Intrinsic Motivation. Plenum Press, New York, 1975
26. Weinberg R: The relationship between extrinsic rewards and intrinsic motivation in sport. p. 177. In Silva J, Weinberg R (eds): Psychological Foundations of Sport. Human Kinetics Publishers, Champaign, 1984
27. Halliwell W: Intrinsic motivation in sport. p. 85. In Straub W (ed): Sport Psychology: An Analysis of Athlete Behavior. Mouvement Publications, Ithaca, 1978
28. Ryan R, Vallerano R, Deci E: Intrinsic motivation in sport: a cognitive evaluation theory interpretation. p. 321. In Straub W, Williams J (eds): Cognitive Sport Psychology. Sport Science Associates, Lansing, 1984
29. Harter S: Effectance motivation reconsidered: toward a developmental model. Hum Dev, 21:34, 1978
30. Deci E, Ryan R: The experimental exploration of intrinsic motivational processes. p. 39. In Berkowitz L (ed): Advances in Experimental Social Psychology. Vol. 13. Academic Press, New York, 1980
31. Locke E, Saari L, Shaw K, Latham G: Goal setting and task performance. Psychol Bull, 90:125, 1981
32. Botterill C: Psychology of coaching. p. 261. In Suinn R (ed): Psychology in Sports: Methods and Applications. Burgess Publications, Minneapolis, 1980
33. Bandura A: Self efficacy: toward a unifying theory of behavioral change. Psychol Rev, 84:191, 1977
34. Bandura A: Self-efficacy mechanism in human agency. Am Psychol, 37:122, 1982
35. Bandura A, Schunk D: Cultivating competence, self-efficacy and intrinsic interest through proximal self-motivation. J Pers Soc Psychol, 36:816, 1982
36. Latham G, Yukl G: A review of research on the application of goal setting in organizations. Acad Manage J, 18:824, 1975
37. Brawley L: Attributions as social cognitions: contemporary perspectives in sport. p. 212. In Straub W, Williams J (eds): Cognitive Sport Psychology. Sport Science Associates, Lansing, 1984
38. Brawley L, Roberts G: Attributions in sport: research foundations, characteristics, and limitations. p. 197. In Silva J, Weinberg R (eds): Psychological Foundations of Sport. Human Kinetics Publishers, Champaign, 1984
39. Rejeski J, Brawley L: Attribution theory in sport: current status and new perspectives. J Sport Psychol, 5:77, 1983
40. Roberts G: Toward a new theory of motivation in sport: the role of perceived ability. p. 214. In Silva J, Weinberg R (eds): Psychological Foundations of Sport. Human Kinetics Publishers, Champaign, 1984
41. Yukelson D, Weinberg R, Jackson A, West S: Attributions and performance: An empirical test of Kukla's theory. J Sport Psychol, 3:46, 1981
42. Egan G: The Skilled Helper. 2nd Ed. Brooks–Cole, Monterey, 1982

43. Yukelson D, Weinberg R, Jackson A, Richardson P: Interpersonal attraction and leadership within collegiate sport teams. J Sport Behav, 6:28, 1983

44. Ouchi W: Theory Z: How American Business Can Meet the Japanese Challenge. Addison–Wesley, Reading, 1981

45. Smith R: Theoretical and treatment approaches to anxiety reduction. p. 157. In Silva J, Weinberg R (eds): Psychological Foundations of Sport. Human Kinetics Publishers, Champaign, 1984

46. Mahoney M: Cognitive skills and athletic performance. p. 11. In Straub W, Williams J (eds): Cognitive Sport Psychology. Sport Science Associates, Lansing, 1984

47. Kirschenbaum, D, Wittrock D: Cognitive–behavioral interventions in sport: a self-regulatory perspective. p. 81. In Silva J, Weinberg R (eds): Psychological Foundations in Sport. Human Kinetics Publishers, Champaign, 1984

48. Borkovek T: Stress management in athletics: an overview of cognitive and physiological techniques. Motor Skills: Theory into Practice 5:45, 1981

49. Benson H: The Relaxation Response. Avon Books, New York, 1976

50. Jacobson E: Progressive Relaxation. University of Chicago Press, Chicago, 1938

51. Wolpe J, Lazarus A: Behavior Therapy Techniques: A Guide to the Treatment of Neurosis. Pergamon, New York, 1966

52. Ravizza K, Rotella R: Cognitive somatic behavioral interventions in gymnastics. p. 25. In Zaichowsky L, Sime W (eds): Stress Management for Sport. AAPHERD, Reston, 1982

53. Nideffer R, Sharpe R: Attention Control Training: How to Get Control of Your Mind Through Total Concentration. Wydon Books, New York, 1978

54. Silva J: Competitive sport environments: performance enhancement through cognitive intervention. Behav Mod, 6:443, 1982

55. Schultz J, Luthe W: Autogenic Training. Grune and Stratton, New York, 1959

56. Zaichowsky L: Biofeedback for self regulation of competitive stress. p. 55. In Zaichowsky L, Sime W (eds): Stress Management for Sport. AAHPERD, Reston, 1982

57. Daniels F, Landers D: Biofeedback and shotting performance: a test of disregulation and systems theory. J Sport Psychol, 3:271, 1981

58. Bloomfield H, Cain M, Jaffe D: Transcendental Meditation: Discovering Inner Energy and Overcoming Stress. Delacorte Press, New York, 1975

59. Suinn R: Imagery in sports. p. 253. In Silva J, Williams J (eds): Cognitive Sport Psychology. Sport Science Associates, Lansing, 1984

60. Weinberg R: Mental preparation strategies. p. 145. In Silva J, Weinberg R (eds): Psychological Foundations of Sport, Champaign, 1984

61. Corbin C: Mental practice. p. 93. In Morgan W (ed): Ergogenic Aids and Muscular Performance. Academic Press, New York, 1972

62. Archterberg G, Lawlis F: Bridges of the Body–Mind: Behavioral Approaches to Health Care. Institute for Personality and Ability Testing, Champaign, 1982

63. Ziegler S: An overview of anxiety management strategies in sport. p. 257. In Straub W (ed): Sport Psychology: An Analysis of Athlete Behavior. Mouvement Publications, Ithaca, 1978

64. Wolpe J: Psychotherapy of Reciprocal Inhibition. Stanford University Press, Stanford, 1958

65. Goldfried M: Systematic desensitization as training in self control. J Consult Clin Psychol, 37:228, 1971

66. Heyman S: Cognitive intervention: theories, applications, and cautions. p. 289. In Straub W, Williams J (eds): Cognitive Sport Psychology. Sport Science Associates, Lansing, 1984

67. Ellis A: Reason and Emotion in Psychotherapy. Lyle Stuart, New York, 1962

68. Meichenbaum D: Cognitive Behavior Modification: An Integrative Approach. Plenum Press, New York, 1977

69. Smith R: Development of an integrated coping response through cognitive–affective stress management training. In Sarason I, Spielberger C (eds): Stress and Anxiety. Vol. 7. Hemisphere, Washington, 1980

70. Yukelson D: Psychological considerations in coaching baseball. p. 471. In Polk R (ed): Baseball Playbook. Mississippi State University, Mississippi State, 1983

71. Meichenbaum D, Turk K: The cognitive–behavioral management of anxiety, anger, and pain. In Davidson P (ed): The Behavioral Management of Anxiety, Depression, and Pain. Bruner–Mazel, New York, 1976

72. Smith R, Ascough J: Induced affect in stress management training. In Burchfield S (ed): Stress, Psychological and Physiological Interaction. Hemisphere, Washington, 1984

73. Spinelli R, Barrios B: Psyching the college athlete: a comprehensive sport psychology training package. p. 344. In Suinn R (ed): Psychology in Sports: Methods and Applications. Burgess, Minneapolis, 1980

74. Kirschenbaum D, Tomarken A: On facing the generalization problem: the study of self-regulatory failure. In Kendall P (ed): Advances in Cognitive Behavioral Research and Therapy. Vol. 1. Academic Press, New York, 1982

10 | Effects of Heat Exposure on the Exercising Adult

Lawrence E. Armstrong
Joseph E. Dziados

PHYSIOLOGICAL RESPONSES TO EXERCISE IN THE HEAT

The heat produced by the muscles of an average-sized, 70-kg person who is exercising moderately at 70 percent of maximal oxygen uptake ($\dot{V}O_2$ MAX), is enough to raise core temperature (Tre) 1.0°C every 5 to 8 minutes if no thermoregulatory mechanisms are activated. This heat load could result in central nervous system dysfunction and eventual death within 15 minutes.[1] Thermoregulatory mechanisms act in concert with the circulatory system, as part of a larger response, dedicated to the maintenance of constant internal body temperature (Tre). Thermoregulation is dependent upon the body's ability to monitor temperature with respect to the environment and to adjust regional blood flow according to the demands imposed by upright posture and exercise, while attempting to maintain fluid balance.

The body monitors temperature with sensitive-free nerve endings located

The views, opinions, and/or findings contained in this report are those of the authors and should not be construed as an official department of the Army position, policy, or decision, unless so designated by other official documentation.

Human subjects participated in these studies after giving their free and informed voluntary consent. Investigators adhered to AR 70-25 and USAMRDC Regulation 70-25 on Use of Volunteers in Research.

in the preoptic area of the hypothalamus and near the skin surface of most of the body.[2,3] These thermoreceptors monitor Tre and skin temperature (Tsk), respectively, and relay this information to the thermoregulatory center, which is also located in the hypothalamus. Numerous experimental observations suggest that the body uses Tsk as an indicator of ambient conditions by combining a weighted average of temperatures from several body sites simultaneously, while "defending" the maintenance of Tre near 37°C by activating thermoregulatory mechanisms.[1,4,5]

A combination of venomotor and vasomotor tone throughout the body governs regional blood flow, heat distribution, and subsequent heat dissipation by radiation and sweating. However, blood flow rates and distribution must change as regional blood flow requirements (especially to muscle and skin) compete with central blood flow (coronary and pulmonary) and splanchnic beds in the viscera (liver, kidneys, and intestines). Generally, during exercise in the heat, a marked increase in blood flow to the active muscles and coronary vessels occurs with maintenance of blood flow to the brain and skin and a decrease in flow to some of the internal organs.[6]

Although it is not possible to determine what relative combination of venomotor and vasomotor tone is responsible for an observed skin blood flow (SkBF) at any given instant, the effects of Tre and Tsk on SkBF can be quantified. The reflex control of SkBF can be approximated by a combination of Tre and Tsk in which Tre is weighted 10 times Tsk.[7] That is, an increase in Tre is considered much more important to the thermoregulatory center than a corresponding increase in Tsk. The body and limbs have an interconnected venous drainage that involves superficial and deep veins, but the superficial veins, with their rich sympathetic innervation, play a larger role in thermoregulation.[8-10] The body can alter SkBF by venoconstriction (which favors heat retention) and by venodilation (which favors heat loss).[11] Both Tsk and Tre determine the degree to which veins will dilate or constrict, but local venous temperature modifies receptivity to this influence.[9,12] Thus, during exercise a rise in Tsk decreases venoconstriction by a direct, local effect of warming on venous smooth muscle and by a central reflex activated by raising body Tsk and Tre.[9,12,13] However, venomotor tone is always greater during upright exercise than during upright rest, thus lowering cutaneous filling rates. Presumably, this makes more central blood volume (CBV) available for cardiac filling and for maintaining cardiac output (Q̇).[7]

Active vasodilation will occur during exercise, not only to the muscle blood vessel beds so that increased oxygen delivery requirements can be met through increased blood flow, but also to the cutaneous blood vessel beds. In fact, 90 to 100 percent of the increase in SkBF that accompanies a rise in Tre during exercise is due to active vasodilation.[14-16] The actual mechanism responsible for this vasodilation is not certain. Apparently, active vasodilation is intimately linked to sweating activity and a functioning sympathetic nervous system, because no active vasodilation is found in individuals with a congenital absence of sweat glands.[14,17] Cutaneous vasodilation can occur in skin arterioles by either central or local heating; however, in vasodilated hyperthermic subjects, skin arterioles will still vasoconstrict by activation of arterial, cardiopulmonary, or postural reflexes.[18,19] This suggests that maintenance of CBV is of prime importance. It is interesting that skin arterioles in the extremities are innervated only by constrictor nerves, and arterioles in most other locations are additionally innervated by dilator nerves.[20] Although the cutaneous arterioles in the hands and feet are not very responsive to baroreflexes (despite only neuroconstrictor innervation), the arterioles of skin in the extremities, muscle, and intestinal vasculature are very involved in the response.[21-24] The response of the skin arterioles depends on local skin temperature (as it is with the venous system) and on the central reflex effect of Tre and Tsk. However, the relationship of SkBF to Tre at a given Tsk is not affected substantially by exercise unless the Tsk is greater than 38°C.[19] Above this temperature, SkBF does not increase proportionally to rising Tre during exercise, probably because of competition between the skin, muscle, and central circulation for available blood volume. It is likely that a progressive rise in SkBF and skin blood volume occurs throughout exercise.[25] In fact, in one study 70 percent of the reduction in stroke volume (SV) during exercise in the heat was accounted for by peripheral pooling.[7] Any regulation of the blood displaced to the skin during upright exercise must occur on the arterial side of the circulation through vasoconstriction.[26] Taken as a whole, it is suggested that Tsk may exert its reflex influence on SkBF by modulating vasoconstrictor outflow, whereas Tre acts mainly on the active vasodilator system.[14]

Since blood flow to inactive skeletal muscle decreases at the onset of exercise and remains decreased, it is apparent that vasoconstrictor outflow to inactive skeletal muscle is maintained or increased throughout exercise, much as it is with splanchnic vasculature. Visceral vasoconstriction is probably mediated by central and cutaneous thermoreceptor monitoring, which in turn causes increased vasoconstriction during exercise in the heat. The question of whether splanchnic venoconstriction occurs during hyperthermia or exercise remains unanswered.[27]

Prolonged, moderately hard exercise in heat results in progressive declines in SV, central venous pressure (CVP), aortic mean pressure (AoMP), and CBV ("cardiovascular drift" phenomenon), while Q stays fairly constant and SkBF continues to rise.[14] When the need for increased SkBF is not met, Tre rises, thereby limiting muscle activity and exercise intensity. There is simply not enough Q or regional blood flow available to raise SkBF to the levels noted during rest.[26] Under these conditions, blood flow to exercising muscle may also be reduced, but this has not been established.[14,28,29]

Sweating occurs when increases in SkBF and radiation are not sufficient to maintain thermal equilibrium. About 3 million sweat glands are present in the skin, varying in number over the body. The face has the greatest density of sweat glands, but the trunk has the greatest absolute number.[30] The number of glands is determined genetically and fixed before birth. Although few differences in the density of sweat glands exist between men and women and among races (and although sweat gland training has been evoked to account for differences in sweating ability), interesting findings regarding sweat gland function have been published recently. In acclimatized men and women, for example, it was reported that women had a higher mean sweating rate per degree of Tre elevation, suggesting that their thermoregulatory mechanism is more sensitive.[31] Also, women were noted to tolerate humid heat better, with superior sweat suppression from skin wettedness, but were found to handle dry heat less well than men.[32]

The majority of sweat glands are eccrine, which are stimulated primarily by thermal stress and secrete a dilute solution. Apocrine sweat glands are located mainly in the axillary and pubic areas and are thought to secrete in response to emotional stress. Sweat secretion is stimulated by release of acetylcholine, mediated through the sympathetic nervous system. It is generally believed that the rate of sympathetic nervous activity (SNA) proportionally governs the rate of secretion. Sweating may occur within 1.5 seconds after initiation of exercise, even prior to any measurable increase in Tre or Tsk.[33] This suggests that the initial response to exercise is neural in nature. However, a prolonged sweating response, unlike the venomotor and vasomotor responses, seems to be unaffected by exercise[7] and depends on Tre and a weighted average of Tsk over the body. The effect of a change in Tre per unit of response is about 10 times that of a similar change in Tsk. Further, an increase in local skin temperature increases the sensitivity of the sweating response to the reflex caused by Tre and Tsk, but in a nonlinear fashion.[34]

The problem of fluid balance during exercise in the heat is compounded by several factors. Normal turnover of water averages about 2 to 2.5 L per day, but during exercise in the heat 10 to 15 L of water loss is not unusual.[30] Sweating obviously leads to fluid loss. Respiratory tract losses, especially in dry, hot climates with low water vapor pressure, can be substantial.[35] As a result of the decrease in visceral blood flow during exercise, water absorption from the intestinal tract may be reduced, although this has not been investigated. Concomitant with the change to an upright posture and subsequently with exercise, a 10 to 15 percent drop in plasma volume can occur in the first 5 to 10 minutes.[36–38] This has the effect of reducing CBV further. Also, progressive dehydration during exercise decreases the sensitivity of the sweating response per unit temperature rise, so that the rate of sweating needed for a given thermal steady state is achieved at an increased Tre.[30] The body can react to some of this loss in CBV by decreasing blood flow to metabolically inactive muscle and diverting blood from the viscera. A decreased blood flow to the kidneys and activation of vasopressin (antidiuretic hormone) helps conserve water and CBV.

In summary, a marked decrease in the CBV occurs during exercise in the heat because a number of simultaneous demands are placed on the circulatory system. High SkBF secondary to high Tre and Tsk causes skin blood volume to increase rapidly to its maximum. The extremities experience a loss of plasma volume to the extravascular space as well as the effect of upright posture and dependent pooling of blood. Combined with arterial vasodilation in the muscle beds and additional fluid losses from sweating, these factors place a severe stress on the body to maintain CBV. Limitation to exercise may result, then, from breakdowns in either the circulatory or the thermoregulatory system. Because of the thermal load from exercise and the environment, the capabilities of the circulatory and thermoregulatory systems may be exceeded; in this case, Tre rises until the individual stops exercising secondary to discomfort or heat illness. Circulatory breakdown is the consequence of an inability to satisfy simultaneous demands for high blood flow to muscle and skin in the face of a reduced CBV. To keep $\dot{Q}$ at the necessary level, heart rate and SV must be maintained, but when venous return and cardiac filling pressure are decreased, SV is also reduced. The arterial baroreflex will increase heart rate (HR) to compensate for the fall in AoMP (caused by decreased $\dot{Q}$) and to attempt to keep $\dot{Q}$ elevated. Breakdown occurs when HR reaches its maximum. This can happen at exercise intensities that are much less than maximal in relatively cool conditions.[30]

PHYSIOLOGY OF HEAT ACCLIMATIZATION AND ACCLIMATION

The physiological adaptations that improve heat tolerance are called heat acclimatization when they result from heat exposure in a natural environment. When they are induced by the artificial climatic stimuli in an environmental chamber, they are called heat acclimation.[39] As the human body adapts to heat, rectal temperature and heart rate decrease while plasma volume and sweat rate increase. The function of these physiological adaptations is to improve heat transfer from the body's core to its periphery and ultimately to the external environment. If heat is not transferred to the surroundings, it may be stored in core areas and work output will be diminished secondary to hyperthermia. Heat acclimatization (HA) and heat acclimation are best achieved by exercising in moderate to hot ambient conditions or by passive heat exposure, for a minimum of 1.5 to 2 hours daily.[40]

Table 10-1 is a summary of many previous HA findings. Each bar represents the number of days of repeated heat exposure needed for that parameter to achieve approximately 95 percent of the maximal response (the "plateau day"). The range of each plateau day cannot be defined more precisely because of interpersonal differences and the variety of environments used in HA studies.

Table 10-1. "Plateau Days" of Physiological Adaptations During Heat Acclimation*

	Days of Heat Acclimatization													
	1	2	3	4	5	6	7	8	9	10	11	12	13	14
Plasma volume expansion			▬	▬	▬	▬								
Heart rate decrease			▬	▬	▬									
Perceived exertion decrease			▬	▬	▬	▬								
Rectal temperature decrease					▬	▬	▬	▬						
Sweat rate increase										▬	▬	▬	▬	▬
Sweat Na+ and Cl− concentration decrease						▬	▬	▬	▬	▬				

* Point at which ≈95% of the response occurs.

Table 10-1 clearly indicates that the systems of the human body respond to thermal stimuli at different rates.

The fainting commonly observed during the first few days of heat exposure indicates that cardiovascular instability may be a problem for the adult who is not accustomed to exercising in the heat. Bean and Eichna,[41] for example, reported that 66 percent of all syncope cases occurred on the first 2 days of work in the heat. The primary cardiovascular adaptation involves an expansion of plasma volume (PV) during the first 3 to 6 days of HA.[42] Because blood must be shared between the skin (for cooling) and the deep working muscles, an increased PV is an advantage during exercise in the heat. This PV expansion has been reported to range from +3 to +27 percent when compared with initial levels.[43] It also may be a transitory state that is followed by a return to preacclimatization levels after other body systems have adapted. A 15 to 25 percent decrease in heart rate accompanies plasma volume expansion[40,44] and typically is attributed to increased cardiac filling pressure and stroke volume with no change in either cardiac output or blood pressure.[45]

The observation of a decreased rectal temperature (Tre) after 3 to 5 days of repeated heat exposure is another hallmark of HA.[44,46] This is significant because an elevated Tre is a limiting factor in exercise performance. Because the maintenance of an elevated Tre appears to be essential for achieving HA successfully,[46] it has been recommended that exercise intensity exceed 50 percent of the person's $\dot{V}O_2$MAX and that increased metabolic heat production is the cause of increased Tre. This means that clothing should be chosen with discrimination during HA. Rubber sweatsuits and insulated garments may cause excessive heat storage. The body's heat dissipation mechanisms must be allowed to function if heat exhaustion and heat stroke are to be avoided.

Improved work efficiency has been observed in a group of subjects who exercised daily in the heat.[47] This means that trained athletes may do the same amount of work, but expend less energy, after HA. This improvement in work efficiency during HA is supported by a reduction in subjective ratings of perceived exertion during exercise.

An individual's initial level of fitness may affect how well he or she tolerates exercise in the heat. In fact, an individual's $\dot{V}O_2MAX$ is significantly related to the number of days required for Tre to plateau and is a primary factor in the maintenance and decay of HA.[48] A high fitness level, gained by training in a cool climate, facilitates performance in the heat but does not replace acclimatization by heat exposure.[46,49] Gisolfi,[50] for example, demonstrated that 8 weeks of interval training in a cool environment produced 50 percent of the total HA response.

After leaving a hot environment to train in cool conditions, an athlete can maintain the benefits of HA for 6 to 28 days,[48,51] depending on the training schedule and the environmental conditions involved. During the decay period, heat tolerance gradually diminishes. One investigation[52] demonstrated that the decay of HA after spending 6 days in a cool environment can be neutralized by training in the heat once per week during a 4-hour intermittent exercise bout.

The biophysical processes that remove heat from the skin include conduction, convection, radiation, and evaporation.[53] Evaporation removes a majority of the heat from the body of an individual who is sweating freely. Typically, the whole body sweat rate increases during HA, allowing more thorough skin wetting and greater evaporative cooling. If sweat rates do not exceed 400 to 600 ml/hour, increases in whole body sweat rate may not be stimulated.[43,44] Although sweat is a dilute mixture of many organic compounds,[54] sodium $(Na+)$ and chloride $(Cl-)$ are the only sweat electrolytes currently known to be altered during the course of HA. Both $Na+$ and $Cl-$ concentrations decrease during chronic heat exposure, whereas magnesium and potassium do not.[43] The conservation of electrolytes during HA, concurrent with an increased sweat rate, offers obvious benefits to an individual working in the heat.

While age appears to have little impact on the rate at which HA is gained,[55] age-related differences in heat tolerance do seem to occur.[56] Age has been recognized as a causal factor in heat stroke, especially in preadolescents and adults older than 40 years of age.[57] The maximal secretory capacity of sweat glands is less in these two groups,[55] even though HA improves thermoregulation at all ages. Whether the decrease in the responsiveness of the sweat glands in older persons is an age-related change or a reflection of their lower $\dot{V}O_2MAX$, is not known.[58]

ASSESSMENT AND EXPRESSION OF ENVIRONMENTAL FACTORS

The nonenvironmental factors governing heat exchange between wet skin and the environment include skin temperature, sweat rate, metabolic heat production, body movements, clothing, and the shape and size of the person. The environmental factors include air temperature, air humidity, radiant energy,

Table 10-2. Heat Stress Indices: 1905 to Present

Name and Abbreviation	Year	Criteria Used	Reference
Wet bulb thermometer (WB)	1905	Wet bulb temperature	60
Effective temperature (ET)	1927	Wet and dry bulb temperature, air movement	61
Predicted 4-hour sweat rate (P4SR)	1947	Air movement, humidity, air temperature, radiant energy, work rate, and clothing	62
Heat stress index (HS)	1955	Evaporative cooling and maximal evaporative cooling and maximal evaporative capacity of the air	63
Wet bulb globe temperature (WBGT)	1957	Temperatures of standard black globe, dry shaded bulb, and wet bulb	64
Discomfort index (DI)	1959	Arithmetic mean of dry and wet bulb temperatures	65
Index of thermal stress (ITS)	1963	Same as HS, plus solar radiation and clothing considerations	66
Oxford index/wet–dry index (WDI)	1963	Wet and dry bulb temperatures	67
Relative heat strain (RHS)	1966	Air temperature, air movement, humidity, work rate, solar radiation, and clothing	68
Wet globe thermometer (WGT)	1971	Air temperature, humidity, air movement, and thermal radiation	69

air movement, and barometric pressure.[53] It would be convenient if all of these factors could be incorporated into one expression so that the effects of any combination of environmental and nonenvironmental factors could be examined. However, it has been recognized for decades that environmental heat factors (stress) must be distinguished from the physiological consequences (strain) that result when a person is exposed to hot environments.[59]

The physiological strain imposed by a given environmental heat stress historically has been evaluated using wet and dry bulb temperatures, air movement, humidity, and solar radiant energy. Many attempts to reduce heat stress to a single expression using these factors have been made, yet no index can accurately express physiological strain for all subjects and work rates. Table 10-2 describes several heat stress indices and details the criteria used to develop them.

The most commonly used heat stress index (HSI) in America today is the wet bulb globe temperature (WBGT) index. It was initially developed for military use and was first utilized at the Marine Corps Recruit Depot, South Car-

Table 10-3. Warnings for Mass Participation Road Races, Based on the WBGT Index

WBGT Reading	Precautions
18–22°C	Runners should monitor themselves closely for signs of impending heat injury and slow running pace as necessary
23–28°C	Runners must slow pace and be very aware of warning signs of heat injury
>28°C	Races should not start under these conditions

(Modified from Hughson RL, Standt LA, Mackie JM: Monitoring road racing in the heat. Phys Sportsmed, 11:94–105, 1983.)

olina, in 1956,[64] with a two-thirds reduction in heat casualties and an increase in effective training time. Since its development, the WBGT index also has been used widely in industry and athletics.[70,71] Three simple observations (Table 10-2) are required to calculate this index: the temperature of a standard black globe thermometer (Tg), the shaded dry bulb temperature (Tdb), and the temperature of a wet bulb thermometer (Twb), which is naturally ventilated and exposed to ambient solar radiation. Outdoor use of the WBGT index consists of a simple weighting of these three temperatures using the following formula:

$$WBGT = (0.7\ Twb) + (0.2\ Tg) + (0.1\ Tdb)$$

For indoor use of the WBGT index, the following formula is used:

$$WBGT = (0.7\ Twb) + (0.3\ Tg)$$

The WBGT exhibits a strong relationship with the wet globe thermometer (WGT); WBGT can be approximated by adding 1°C to the WGT reading.[72] The WBGT also is strongly correlated with the DI, the HSI used in Israel (E. Sohar, personal communication, 1983).[65] Because the WBGT includes no measurement of air movement, it is not applicable to all hot environments. It is most useful in a band of conditions where the heat stress reaches a critical physiological strain level and heat exhaustion and heat stroke are most likely to occur.[53]

A variety of devices have been used to measure the WBGT and WGT indices. The original WBGT readings were taken by simple thermometers.[64] Modern heat stress monitors and WBGT meters are available (Reuter Stokes, Cambridge, Ontario, Canada) in forced convection or naturally ventilated models. These devices allow separation of Twb, Tdb, and Tg values. Collection of WGT readings has been simplified by the development of the Botsball thermometer (Howard Engineering Co., Bethlehem, PA).

The most common use for any HSI in sports is to set limits above which certain precautions should be observed. These precautions include time of exposure to hot environments, work intensity/duration, fluid replacement, heat illness surveillance, and increased air movement. For example, the WBGT index recently has been used to establish warnings for mass-participation road races in an attempt to prevent runners from collapsing with heat injury.[70] These precautions are described in Table 10-3. Industrial WBGT limits have been set

Table 10-4. U.S. Army Guidelines for Work/Rest Cycles and
Water Intake, Based on the WGT Index

WGT Reading (°C)	Water Intake (L/hour)	Work/Rest Cycle (minutes)
<26.7	0.0–0.5	50/10
26.7–28.3	0.5–1.0	50/10
28.3–30.0	1.0–1.5	45/15
30.0–31.1	1.5–2.0	30/30
>31.1	2.0	20/40

(Modified from U.S. Department of the Army: Prevention of
Heat Injury. Washington D.C., 1982, Circular No. 40-82-3.)

by the Occupational Safety Health Administration of the U.S. Department of Labor[73] for light, moderate, and heavy work loads.

The U.S. Army has utilized the WGT index to establish guidelines for work/rest cycles and water intake.[74] Military units observe the guidelines that appear in Table 10-4. These WGT values apply to persons wearing lightweight clothing; approximately 10°C should be added to the measured WGT reading to establish guidelines for persons wearing impermeable clothing, such as raincoats or rubberized suits. Recent findings at this laboratory indicate that WGT readings can underestimate WBGT temperatures by 8 to 11° F, under conditions of low humidity and high wind speed (WT Matthew, unpublished observation). WGT limits have been established for industrial settings by the American Industrial Hygiene Association.[75]

Although idealistic, the "perfect" HSI should: accurately predict physiological strain over a wide range of environmental conditions; account for a wide range of individual differences in the response to thermal stress; include all of the important variables (Table 10-2) that affect the heat balance of the body; and be simple enough for everyday use.[39,40–42] None of the HSI in Table 10–2 meets all of these criteria, because they were designed for specific purposes (e.g., industry, military). Therein may lie the key to the most appropriate use of HSI. Rather than selecting the best index for all uses, one should select the index that best predicts thermal stress for a known set of circumstances.

HEAT ILLNESS

Heat illness involves a spectrum of symptoms resulting from the physiological toll of maintaining normal body temperature in the face of a large environmental or metabolic heat load.[76] Symptoms are manifest as regulatory mechanisms begin to fail. A great deal of variation exists in susceptibility to heat illness,[77] but certain susceptible individuals and predisposing factors can be identified.

Elderly persons are more susceptible to heat illness, probably because they do not sense temperature changes as readily. They also tend to have less cardiovascular reserve than younger persons. Although not of immediate concern to sports medicine staff members, infants are more heat-labile because of the immaturity of their thermoregulatory system.[78] Athletes are quite vulnerable to heat illness; in fact, heat illness is the second leading cause of death among young athletes in the United States.[79]

A number of predisposing factors or diseases increase the likelihood of heat injury. Any disease that substantially affects the cardiovascular system will limit heat tolerance. One example is any type of heart disease (congestive, ischemic, arteriosclerotic, or hypertensive); since the circulatory system is intimately linked with the thermoregulatory system, any body fluid disturbance (especially dehydration in excess of 3 percent) can be important.[76] Increased endogenous heat load is also a risk factor; any infectious state with fever, delirium tremens, seizures, psychosis, or ingestion of amphetamine-like drugs may be deleterious.[76] Abnormalities of the skin or sweat gland function interfere with heat dissipation, hence burns, heat rash, sunburn, scleroderma, and cystic fibrosis can cause problems. Anticholinergic drugs (including antidepressants, antihistamines, antispasmodics, and antipsychotics) can depress sweating. Alcohol, which causes peripheral vasodilation and is also a diuretic, may have a dual adverse effect, causing absorption of ambient heat load through vasodilation (only when Tsk is greater than ambient temperature) and increased dehydration through increased urination. Lack of acclimatization affects susceptibility. Clothing, which affects ability to dissipate heat, and conditions such as fatigue and lack of sleep also have been implicated in heat illness.[80] Previous episodes of heat stroke in an individual predispose to heat injury.[81]

The spectrum of heat illness ranges from "prickly heat" to heat stroke, the former being a nuisance and the latter being a life-threatening emergency. The self-limiting, minor illnesses are not discussed.

Heat cramps occur most commonly in the more active muscle groups (usually the calves) in fit, acclimatized individuals. It is not clear what causes heat cramps; it is interesting that serum electrolytes are normal.[76] The most effective treatment for heat cramps is saline solution administered either orally or intravenously. If given orally, the concentration should be about 0.1 percent (the equivalent of ¼ teaspoon of salt in 1 quart of water). Salt tablets should not be taken because they can cause nausea, vomiting, and exacerbate dehydration. Heat cramps are quickly relieved by this treatment and have no lasting effect.

Heat exhaustion is a vaguely defined syndrome that can occur in anyone exposed to heat stress. General symptoms include headache, giddiness, anorexia, nausea, vomiting, malaise, thirst, muscle cramps, tetany (from hyperventilation), orthostasis, tachycardia, and syncope. Sweating is always present. Temperature may be normal or only moderately elevated (although temperatures up to 39.5°C have been reported). Irritability, anxiety, slight confusion, and slight impairment of judgment are also common. In these regards, heat exhaustion is distinguished from heat stroke by the milder impairment of temperature regulation and mental function. Grossly psychotic behavior, seizures, and coma, which are common with heat stroke, are not present in heat exhaustion.

Two types of heat exhaustion occur: that primarily due to water loss and that primarily due to salt depletion. Usually, a combined form is observed. Water-depletion heat exhaustion tends to occur in less than 3 days, whereas predominantly salt-depletion exhaustion usually develops over a period longer than 3 days. A precise distinction may not be important because treatment is similar for both deficiencies. No actual cellular damage occurs in heat exhaustion; liver and muscle enzymes are normal. This contrasts with heat stroke, in which serum enzyme levels are universally elevated. Apparently, there is a small subgroup of individuals (usually athletes) who exhibit high temperatures, hypotension, and confusion, yet experience a heat illness that lies somewhere between exhaustion and stroke. For this reason, the individual should be treated for the more severe possibility if there is doubt. Treatment consists of rest in a cool environment, the replacement of fluids orally for mild cases of heat exhaustion, and intravenous replacement for more severe cases or if nausea and vomiting limit oral intake. Dehydration is very common and can require up to 4 L of fluid administration over a 6-hour period. If spontaneous cooling does not occur, heat stroke may evolve. Following therapy, individuals usually recover within 12 hours and experience no sequelae.[76]

Because heat stroke is the most serious heat illness, with mortality rates of 10 to 80 percent, it presents a true medical emergency. Heat stroke, unlike heat cramps, heat exhaustion, and other self-limiting heat illnesses, is hall-marked by a loss of thermoregulatory capacity. Individuals can have a Tre over 45°C, with elevations to 41°C quite common. However, since heat exhaustion temperatures of up to 39.5°C have been reported, there is no specific, single diagnostic Tre by which to identify heat stroke. The central nervous system (CNS) is probably the organ system most sensitive to temperature changes. Early CNS dysfunction may be manifested as irritability, poor judgment, and bizarre behavior and eventually may lead to psychosis, seizures, and coma. The diagnosis of heat stroke requires evidence of major alteration of consciousness or severe confusion.[76]

The two types of heat stroke are classic (CHS) and exertional (EHS). CHS is more common in the elderly, the ill, and infants. Since CHS evolves over several days of heat stress, individuals may become significantly dehydrated and anhydrosis may occur. CHS symptoms initially include chills, throbbing pressure in the head, nausea, unsteadiness, and piloerection on the chest and upper arms,[76] which progress rapidly to bizarre behavior or collapse. While sweating may be present or absent in either CHS or EHS, tachycardia is always present, as is hyperventilation (both serving to increase heat loss). EHS, on the other hand, usually occurs in fit and motivated individuals, especially when they are unacclimatized.[82] EHS tends to develop in a few hours, not allowing time for severe dehydration to occur; thus 50 percent of individuals with EHS sweat profusely.

The treatment of heat stroke as a medical emergency in the hospital is beyond the scope of this discussion. In the field, however, cooling should be instituted immediately if the temperature is greater than 41°C. The more rapid the cooling, the lower the mortality.[83] If heat stroke is suspected, clothing should be removed from the victim and cool liquids, ice, or a fine-mist spray applied to the skin. The prognosis for heat stroke is worse if the victim becomes unconscious and then depends on the duration of coma. If coma lasts less than

3 to 4 hours, a good outcome is likely. If the coma persists for more than 10 hours, the victim probably will die.[84] Because of the potentially serious outcome, the best solution for heat stroke and for any heat illness is prevention.

Prevention of Heat Illness

Heat stroke and heat exhaustion occur most often when intense work is performed in hot environments. Young, fit individuals are especially vulnerable to heat injury because athletic competition, pride, ambition, or discipline drive them to produce large quantities of metabolic heat. In fact, the probability of becoming a heat casualty can be significantly reduced for these individuals if the causes of heat illness are understood and if preventive measures are taken.

Persons who know that they are heat-intolerant or possess factors that predispose them to heat injury should take the necessary precautions to avoid dehydration and elevated Tre during exercise. All persons should monitor WBGT readings during exercise. Also, athletes should train during the cooler hours of the day and should wear loose-fitting, lightweight clothing to encourage evaporative cooling.

The most important factor in the short-term (less than 3 days) prevention of hyperthermia is adequate hydration. The old myth that "limited drinking toughens athletes" is not supported by either medical records or practical experience. No scientific evidence exists to show that the human body can adapt to long-term dehydration. Because sweat is mostly water, hemoconcentration occurs when fluid losses result from heavy sweating. Thus the immediate requirement of the adult exercising in heat is water, not electrolyte supplementation. Unfortunately, thirst will not begin to stimulate increased drinking until body weight losses reach 1 to 2 percent of the initial body weight (0.75 to 1.5 L). Although voluntary intake of water can be improved by cooling and flavoring water supplies,[85] only one half to two thirds of the fluid lost in sweat and urine will be replaced, because the thirst mechanism is not an adequate indicator of the body's water needs. This is significant because strength, endurance, circulatory function, mental performance, and thermoregulation are impaired when body weight losses exceed 3 to 5 percent.[85,86] A 6- to 10-percent body weight loss is associated with vertigo, cyanosis, dyspnea, and spasticity. The lethal hypohydration range is reported to be -15 to -25 percent of initial body weight.[85]

The replacement of fluid losses during exercise is limited by the thoroughness and efficiency of gastric emptying (GE). If the contents of the stomach do not enter the intestines, the cardiovascular system and working muscles cannot benefit fully from ingested fluids. The research of Costill and Saltin[88] indicates that GE during rest and exercise may be retarded by at least four factors. First, exercise has no effect on GE until the intensity exceeds 70 percent $\dot{V}O_{2MAX}$, but exercise intensities in excess of 70 percent of $\dot{V}O_{2MAX}$ are commonly reported,[89] even during distance races as long as a marathon (42.2 km). Also, the composition of a fluid retards GE if: (1) the temperature is greater than 15 to 20°C; (2) the volume consumed is less than 600 ml; and (3) the glucose concentration exceeds 139 mmol/L. These findings underscore the benefits of using large volumes of cool, dilute solutions as replacement drinks during exercise. Cool, pure water is the drink of choice in most instances.

The long-term (3 days or more) prevention of heat exhaustion and heat stroke also involves electrolyte deficits secondary to sweat and urinary losses. Most electrolyte deficiency research[54,90] has focused on Na+, Cl−, and potassium (K+) losses. Hubbard and colleagues[90] recently reviewed the literature regarding long-term salt and water deficits. They concluded that previous sodium chloride (NaCl) intake recommendations for continuous desert living (15 to 30 g/day) may be unnecessarily high in light of hormonal adaptations (aldosterone) during HA that result in NaCl conservation in urine and sweat.[91] The individuals most likely to suffer serious electrolyte deficits are unacclimatized persons during the first 3 to 5 days of continuous heat exposure.[90] For the professional or recreational athlete living in the United States, liberal salting of meals provides adequate dietary NaCl intake for nearly all exercise-induced electrolyte losses incurred during hot weather training. Long-term K+ depletion is possible during extended desert living,[92] but for nearly all individuals involved in sports in North America, the U.S. minimum daily recommended intake of K+ (2.0 to 3.9 g/day) is adequate to maintain a positive K+ balance.[43]

The intensity and duration of certain competitive events require that precautions be taken when environmental heat stress is great. Distance cycling and marathon running in the heat, for example, superimpose a large metabolic heat production on environmental heat stress. We observed a world-class distance runner before and during the 1984 Olympic marathon who exhibited a prolific sweating rate (3.71 L/hour) and lost 5.43 kg (−8.1 percent) body weight during his 134-minute race. Because his gastric emptying during the race was estimated at 1 L/hour,[88] he could not ingest water faster than 1 L/hour, so large body water deficits were inevitable. Fluid losses secondary to sweating typically exceed water intake during marathons, and body weight losses of 1.0 to 5.9 kg are not uncommon.[93] Postmarathon Tre values exceeding 40°C also are frequently reported.[89,93] It must be concluded, therefore, that certain athletic events are inherently likely to predispose athletes to heat illness. The only means of preventing heat injury may be to postpone the event or to schedule it during cool conditions.[94] It is unlikely that highly competitive athletes will limit performance voluntarily.

SUMMARY

Exercise in the heat may place severe demands on the circulatory and thermoregulatory systems. Blood volume must be distributed between visceral, cutaneous, muscular, and cardiopulmonary blood vessel beds according to regional and central blood flow requirements. Sweating augments the removal of heat and is facilitated by increased cutaneous flow. Heat acclimatization and acclimation occur primarily from greater sweat rate and increased blood volume, which result in improved heat dissipation. HA may be facilitated by repeated exposures to the heat while exercising at greater than 50 percent V̇O₂MAX. Although many heat stress indices are available, the exercising adult should be aware that no one index is ideal. A HSI should be selected to match the intended activity, such as the WBGT index for runners in road races. Since heat illness can be lethal, emphasis should be placed on prevention. Prevention can be optimized by careful consideration of environmental conditions, proper dress, liberal consumption of fluids, and prior HA. Even when these factors are considered, the intensity of exercise should be reduced during conditions of severe heat stress. Unfortunately, competitive athletes are not likely to observe this precaution. Sponsors of competitive events held during hot weather must be prepared to adjust or even cancel events for the safety of all participants.

REFERENCES

1. Nadel ER: A brief overview. p.1. In Nadel ER (ed): Problems with Temperature Regulation during Exercise. Academic Press, New York, 1977
2. Hensel H, Iggo A, Witt I: A quantitative study of sensitive cutaneous thermoreceptors with C afferent fibers. J Physiol 153:113, 1960
3. Nakayama T, Hammel HT, Hardy JD, Eisenman JS: Thermal stimulation and electrical activity of single units of the preoptic region. Am J Physiol 204:1122, 1963
4. Saltin B, Hermansen L: Esophageal, rectal, and muscle temperature during exercise. J Appl Physiol 21:1757, 1966
5. Wyndham CH: The physiology of exercise under heat stress. Ann Rev Physiol 35:193, 1973
6. Mitchell JH, Blomqvist G: Maximal oxygen intake. N Engl J Med 284:1018, 1971
7. Wenger CB: Circulatory and sweating responses during exercise and heat stress. In Adair ER (ed): Microwaves and Thermoregulation. Academic Press, New York, 1983
8. Webb–Peploe MM, Shepherd JT: Responses of large hindlimb veins of the dog to sympathetic nerve stimulation. Am J Physiol 215:299, 1968
9. Webb–Peploe MM, Shepherd JT: Responses of dogs' cutaneous veins to local and central temperature changes. Circ Res 23:693, 1968
10. Thauer R: Circulatory adjustments to climatic requirements. In Hamilton WF, Dow P (eds): Handbook of Physiology. 2nd Ed. Vol. 3. American Physiological Society, Washington, D.C. 1965
11. Goetz RH: Effect of changes in posture on peripheral circulation, with special reference to skin temperature readings and the plethysmogram. Circulation, 1:56, 1950
12. Rowell LB, Brengelmann GL, Detry JMR, Wyss C: Venomotor responses to local and remote thermal stimuli to skin in exercising man. J Appl Physiol 30:72, 1971
13. Vanhoutte PM: Physical factors of regulation. p. 443. In Bohr DF, Somlyo Ap, Sparks HV, Jr. (eds): Handbook of Physiology. 2nd Ed. Vol. 2. American Physiological Society, Washington, D.C., 1980
14. Rowell LB: Cardiovascular aspects of human thermoregulation. Circ Res 52:367, 1983
15. Greenfield ADM: The circulation through the skin. p. 1325. In Hamilton WF, Dow P (eds): Handbook of Physiology. 2nd Ed. Vol. 2. American Physiological Society, Washington, D.C., 1963

16. Shepherd JT: Physiology of the Circulation in Human Limbs in Health and Disease. WB Saunders, Philadelphia, 1963
17. Brengelmann GL, Freund PR, Rowell LB et al: Absence of active cutaneous vasodilation associated with congenital absence of sweat glands in man. Am J Physiol 240:H571, 1981
18. Crossley RJ, Greenfield ADM, Plassaras GC, Stephens D: The interrelation of thermoregulatory and baroreceptor reflexes in the control of blood vessels in the human forearm. J Physiol 183:628, 1966
19. Johnson JM, Rowell LB, Brengelmann GL: Modification of the skin blood flow–body temperature relationship by upright exercise. J Appl Physiol 37:880, 1974
20. Fox RH, Edholm OG: Nervous control of the cutaneous circulation. Br Med Bull 19:110, 1963
21. Rowell LB, Wyss CR, brengelmann GL: Sustained human skin and muscle vasoconstriction with reduced baroreceptor activity. J Appl Physiol 34:639, 1973
22. McNamara HI, Sikorski JM, Clavin H: The effects of lower body negative pressure on hand blood flow. Cardiovasc Res 3:284, 1969
23. Beiser GD, Zelis R, Epstein SE et al: The role of skin and muscle resistance vessels in reflexes mediated by the baroreceptor system. J Clin Invest 49:225, 1970
24. Rowell LB, Detry JMR, Blackmon HR, Wyss C: Importance of the splanchnic vascular bed in human blood pressure regulation. J Appl Physiol 32:213, 1972
25. Ekelund LG: Circulatory and respiratory adaptation during prolonged exercise. Acta Physiol Scand, 70: suppl. 292, 5–38, 1967
26. Rowell LB: Competition between skin and muscle. In Nadel ER (ed): Problems with Temperature Regulation during Exercise. Academic Press, New York, 1977
27. Ludbrook J, Faris IB, Iannos J et al: Lack of effect of isometric handgrip exercise on the responses of the carotid sinus baroreceptor reflex in man. Clin Sci Mol Med 55:189, 1978
28. Detry JMR, Brengelmann GL, Rowell LB, Wyss C: Skin and muscle components of forearm blood flow in directly heated resting man. J Appl Physiol 32:506, 1972
29. Johnson JM, Brengelmann GL, Rowell LB: Interactions between local and reflex influences on human forearm skin blood flow. J Appl Physiol 41:826, 1976
30. Nadel ER: Temperature regulation. p. 130. In Strauss RH (ed): Sports Medicine and Physiology. WB Saunders, Philadelphia, 1979
31. Horstman DH, Christensen E: Acclimatization to dry heat: active men vs active women. J Appl Physiol 52:825, 1982
32. Shapiro Y, Pandolf KB, Avellini BA et al: Physiological responses of men and women to humid and dry heat. J Appl Physiol 42:1, 1980
33. van Beaumont W, Bullard RW: Sweating: its rapid response to muscular work. Science 141:643, 1963
34. Brengelmann GL: Control of sweating rate and skin blood flow during exercise. In Nadel ER (ed): Problems with Temperature Regulation during Exercise. Academic Press, New York, 1977
35. Mitchell JW, Nadel ER, Stolwijk JAJ: Respiratory weight loss during exercise. J Appl Physiol 32:474, 1972
36. Costill DL, Branam L, Eddy D, Fink W: Alterations in red cell volume following exercise and dehydration. J Appl Physiol 37:912, 1974
37. Costill DL, Fink WJ: Plasma volume changes following exercise and thermal dehydration. J Appl Physiol 37:521, 1974
38. Greenleaf JE, Convertino VA, Stremel RW et al: Plasma sodium, calcium, and volume shifts and thermoregulation during exercise in man. J Appl Physiol 43:1026, 1977

39. Bligh J, Johnson KG: Glossary of terms for thermal physiology. J Appl Physiol 35:941, 1973
40. Lind AR, Bass DE: Optimal exposure time for development of acclimatization to heat. Fed Proc 22:704, 1963
41. Bean WB, Eichna LW: Performance in relation to environmental temperature. Fed Proc 2:144, 1943
42. Senay L, Mitchell D, Wyndham CH: Acclimatization in a hot, humid environment: body fluid adjustments. J Appl Physiol 40:786, 1976
43. Armstrong LE, Costill DL, Fink WJ et al: Effects of dietary sodium on body and muscle potassium during heat acclimation. Eur J Appl Physiol, 1985 (in press)
44. Sciaraffa D, Fox SC, Stockmann R, Greenleaf JE: Human Acclimation and Acclimatization to Heat: A Compendium of Research—1968–1978. NASA, Moffett Field, CA, (Technical Memorandum 81181) 1980
45. Rowell LB: Human cardiovascular adjustments to exercise and thermal stress. Physiol Rev 54:75, 1974
46. Pandolf KB: Effects of physical training and cardiorespiratory physical fitness on exercise heat tolerance: recent observations. Med Sci Sports 11:60, 1979
47. Senay L, Kok R: Effects of training and heat acclimatization on blood plasma contents of exercising men. J Appl Physiol 43:591, 1977
48. Pandolf K, Burse RL, Goldman RF: Role of physical fitness in heat acclimation, decay and reintroduction. Ergonomics 20:399, 1977
49. Strydom NB: Comparison of oral and rectal temperature during work in the heat. J Appl Physiol 8:406, 1956
50. Gisolfi CV, Robinson SR: Relationships between physical training, acclimatization and heat tolerance. J Appl Physiol 25:586, 1968
51. Adams JM, Fox RH, Grimby G et al: Acclimatization to heat and its rate of decay in man. J Physiol 152:26, 1960
52. Wyndham CH, Jacobs GE: Loss of acclimatization after six days in cool conditions on the surface of a mine. J Appl Physiol 11:197, 1957
53. Kerslake DM: The Stress of Hot Environments. Cambridge University Press, London, 1972
54. Robinson S, Robinson AH: Chemical composition of sweat. Physiol Rev 34:202, 1954
55. Wagner JA, Robinson S, Tozankoff P, Marino RP: Heat tolerance and acclimatization to work in the heat in relation to age. J Appl Physiol 33:616, 1972
56. Robinson S, Belding HS, Consolazio FC et al: Acclimatization of older men to work in the heat. J Appl Physiol 20:583, 1965
57. Strydom NB: Age as a causal factor in heat stroke. J S Afr Inst Min Metall 72:112, 1971
58. Drinkwater BL, Horvath SM: Heat tolerance and aging. Med Sci Sports 11:49, 1979
59. Lee DK: Seventy-five years of searching for a heat index. Environ Res 22:331, 1980
60. Haldane JS: Influence of high temperature. J Hyg 5:40, 1905
61. Yaglou CP: Temperature, humidity, and air movement in industries: the effective temperature index. J Ind Hyg 9:297, 1927
62. McArdle B, Dunham W, Hollong HE et al: The Prediction of the Physiological Effects of Warm and Hot Environments. Medical Research Council, London, 1947 (No. RNP 47/391)
63. Belding HS, Hatch TF: Index for evaluating heat stress in terms of the resulting physiological strain. Heat Piping Air Cond 27:129, 1955

64. Yaglou CP, Minard D: Control of heat casualties at military training centers. Arch Ind Hlth 16:302, 1957

65. Sohar E: Determination and presentation of heat load in physiologically meaningful terms. Int J Biometeorol 7:22, 1980

66. Givoni B: Estimation of the Effect of Climate on Man: Development of a New Thermal Index. Institute of Technology, Haifa, Israel, 1963 (Research report to UNESCO)

67. Lind AR: Assessment of physiological severity of hot climates. J Appl Physiol 11:35, 1957

68. Lee DK, Henschel A: Effects of physiological and clinical factors on response to heat. Ann NY Acad Sci 134:743, 1966

69. Botsford JH: A wet globe thermometer for environmental heat measurement. Am Ind Hyg Assoc J 32:1, 1971

70. Hughson RL, Standt LA, Mackie JM: Monitoring road racing in the heat. Phys Sportsmed 11:94, 1983

71. Jones RD: Effects of Thermal Stress on Human Performance: A Review and Critique of Existing Methodology. U.S. Army, Aberdeen, NM, 1970 (Technical Memo No. 11-70)

72. Ciriello VM, Snook SM: The prediction of WBGT from the Botsball. Am Ind Hyg Assoc J 38:6,7, 1977

73. Occupational Safety and Health Administration: Recommendations for a Standard for Work in Hot Environments. U.S. Department of Labor, Standards Advisory Committee on Heat, Washington, D.C., 1974

74. U.S. Department of the Army: Prevention of Heat Injury. Washington, D.C., 1982 (Circular No. 40-82-3)

75. American Industrial Hygiene Association: Heating and Cooling for Man in Industry. Akron, OH, 1974

76. Callaham ML: Emergency management of heat illness. p.1. In Emergency Physician Series. Abbott Labs, Chicago, 1979

77. Kew MC: Temperature regulation in heat stroke in man. Isr J Med Sci, 12:759, 1976

78. Schoenfeld Y, Udassin R: Age and sex difference in response to short exposure to extremely dry heat. J Appl Physiol 44:1, 1978

79. Knochel JP: Dog days and siriasis: how to kill a football player. JAMA 233:513, 1975

80. Department of Army, Navy, and Air Force Technical Bulletin: Etiology, prevention, diagnosis, and treatment of adverse effects of heat. Publication No. TB Med 507, p.1. July, 1980

81. Shapiro Y, Magazanik A, Udassin R et al: Heat intolerance in former heat stroke patients. Ann Intern Med 90:913, 1979

82. Costrini AM, Pitt HA, Gustafson AB et al: Cardiovascular and metabolic manifestations of heat stroke and severe heat exhaustion. Am J Med, 66:296, 1979

83. Bynum GP, Patton J, Bowers W et al: Peritoneal lavage cooling in an anesthetized dog heat stroke model. Aviat Space Environ Med 49:779, 1978

84. Shepard RJ, Kavanagh T: Fluid and mineral needs of middle-aged and post-coronary runners. Phys Sportsmed, 6:90, 1978

85. Adolf EF: Physiology of Man in the Desert. Interscience, New York, 1947

86. Herbert WG: Water and electrolytes. pp. 56. In Williams M (ed): Ergogenic Aids in Sport. Human Kinetics Publishers, Champaign, IL, 1983

87. Sawka MN, Francesconi RP, Young AJ et al: Influence of hydration level and body fluids on exercise performance in the heat. JAMA 252:1165, 1984

88. Costill DL, Saltin B: Factors limiting gastric emptying during rest and exercise. J Appl Physiol 37:679, 1974
89. Costill DL: Physiology of marathon running. JAMA 221:1024, 1972
90. Hubbard RW, Armstrong LE, Evans PK, Deluca J: Long-term Water and Salt Deficits: A Military Perspective. Milit Med, 1986 (in press)
91. Conn JW: Acclimatization to heat. Adv Intern Med 3:377, 1949
92. Knochel JP, Vertel RM: Salt loading as a possible factor in the production of potassium deficiency, rhabdomyolysis, and heat injury. Lancet 1:659, 1967
93. Pugh LGCE, Corbett JL, Johnson RL: Rectal temperatures, weight losses, and sweat rates in marathon running. J Appl Physiol 23:347, 352, 1967
94. American College of Sports Medicine: Position stand on prevention of thermal injuries during distance running. Sport Med Bull 19:8, 1984

Index

Page numbers followed by *f* represent figures; numbers followed by *t* represent tables.